Underground Clinical Vignettes

Obstetrics and Gynecology

FOURTH EDITION

Sandra I. Kim, M.D., Ph.D.
Resident in Internal Medicine
Beth Israel Deaconess Medical Center
Harvard Medical School
Boston, Massachusetts

Todd A. Swanson, M.D., Ph.D.
Resident in Radiation Oncology
William Beaumont Hospital
Royal Oak, Michigan

Ronald C. Chen, M.D.
Resident in Radiation Oncology
Harvard Radiation Oncology Program
Harvard Medical School
Boston, Massachusetts

Wolters Kluwer | Lippincott Williams & Wilkins
Health

Philadelphia · Baltimore · New York · London
Buenos Aires · Hong Kong · Sydney · Tokyo

Acquisitions Editor: Nancy Anastasi Duffy
Developmental Editor: Nancy Hoffmann
Managing Editor: Kelly Horvath
Production editor: Kevin Johnson
Marketing manager: Jennifer Kuklinski
Designer: Doug Smock
Compositor: International Typesetting and Composition

© 2008 by Lippincott Williams & Wilkins
UCV Step 2 Emergency Medicine, 3e, 2005 Blackwell Publishers.
Lippincott Williams & Wilkins, a Wolters Kluwer business.

351 West Camden Street   530 Walnut Street
Baltimore, MD 21201   Philadelphia, PA 19106

9 8 7 6 5 4 3 2 1

Library of Congress Cataloging-in-Publication Data
Kim, Sandra.
    Obstetrics and gynecology / Sandra I. Kim, Todd A. Swanson, Ronald Chen. — 4th ed.
        p. ; cm. — (Underground clinical vignettes)
    Includes index.
    Rev. ed. of: Obstetrics and gynecology / Vikhas Bhushan . . . [et al.]. 3rd ed. c2005.
    ISBN-13: 978-0-7817-6840-5
    ISBN-10: 0-7817-6840-3
    1. Gynecology—Case studies.   2. Obstetrics—Case studies.   3. Physicians—
Licenses—United States—Examinations—Study guides.   I. Swanson, Todd A.
II. Chen, Ronald.   III. Obstetrics and gynecology.   IV. Title.   V. Series.
    [DNLM: 1. Genital Diseases, Female—Case Reports.   2. Genital
Diseases, Female—Problems and Exercises.   3. Pregnancy
Complications—Case Reports.   4. Pregnancy Complications—Problems and
Exercises. WP 18.2 K49o 2007]
    RG106.B48 2007
    618'.076—dc22   2007024878

DISCLAIMER

Care has been taken to confirm the accuracy of the information present and to describe generally accepted practices. However, the authors, editors, and publisher are not responsible for errors or omissions or for any consequences from application of the information in this book and make no warranty, expressed or implied, with respect to the currency, completeness, or accuracy of the contents of the publication. Application of this information in a particular situation remains the professional responsibility of the practitioner; the clinical treatments described and recommended may not be considered absolute and universal recommendations.

The authors, editors, and publisher have exerted every effort to ensure that drug selection and dosage set forth in this text are in accordance with the current recommendations and practice at the time of publication. However, in view of ongoing research, changes in government regulations, and the constant flow of information relating to drug therapy and drug reactions, the reader is urged to check the package insert for each drug for any change in indications and dosage and for added warnings and precautions. This is particularly important when the recommended agent is a new or infrequently employed drug.

Some drugs and medical devices presented in this publication have Food and Drug Administration (FDA) clearance for limited use in restricted research settings. It is the responsibility of the health care provider to ascertain the FDA status of each drug or device planned for use in their clinical practice.

To purchase additional copies of this book, call our customer service department at **(800) 638-3030** or fax orders to **(301) 223-2320**. International customers should call **(301) 223-2300**.

Visit Lippincott Williams & Wilkins on the Internet: http://www.lww.com. Lippincott Williams & Wilkins customer service representatives are available from 8:30 am to 6:00 pm, EST.

Underground Clinical Vignettes

Obstetrics and Gynecology

FOURTH EDITION

dedications

Dedicated to the patients we care for.

preface

First published in 1999, the Underground Clinical Vignettes series has provided thousands of students with a highly effective review tool as they prepare for medical examinations, particularly the USMLE Step 1 and 2 examinations. Designed as a quick study guide, each UCV book contains patient-centered clinical cases that highlight a range of medical diagnoses.

With this new edition of Step 2 Underground Clinical Vignettes, we have incorporated feedback from medical students across the country to provide updated cases with expanded treatment and discussion sections. Every title has more cases, drawing from a broader area within each discipline. A new two-page format enables readers to formulate an initial diagnosis prior to reading the answer to each case. The inclusion of relevant magnetic resonance images, radiographs, and photographs allows students to more readily visualize the physical presentation of each case. Breakout boxes, tables, and algorithms have been added, along with twenty all-new board-format questions-and-answers, making this edition of UCV an ideal source of information for examination review, classroom discussion, and clinical rotations.

The clinical vignettes in this Step 2 series have been revised and updated to reflect current medical thinking on medication, pathogenesis, epidemiology, management, and complications. Although each case presents most of the signs, symptoms, and diagnostic findings for a particular illness, patients typically will not present with such a "complete" picture either clinically or on a medical examination. Cases are not meant to simulate a potential real patient or an examination vignette.

Access to LWW's online companion site, ThePoint, will be offered as a premium with the purchase of the Underground Clinical Vignettes Step 2 bundle. Benefits include an online test link and 160 additional new board-format questions covering all UCV subject areas.

We hope you will find the Underground Clinical Vignettes series informative and useful. We welcome any feedback, suggestions, or corrections you have about this series. Please contact us at LWW.com/medstudent.

contributors

Series Editors

Sandra I. Kim, M.D., Ph.D.
Resident in Internal Medicine
Beth Israel Deaconess Medical Center
Harvard Medical School
Boston, Massachusetts

Todd A. Swanson, M.D., Ph.D.
Resident in Radiation Oncology
William Beaumont Hospital
Royal Oak, Michigan

Contributing Editors

Andrew Z. Wang, M.D.
Resident in Radiation Oncology
Harvard Radiation Oncology Program
Harvard Medical School
Boston, Massachusetts

Melody Y. Hou, M.D.
Fellow in Family Planning
Brigham and Women's Hospital
Harvard Medical School
Boston, Massachusetts

Holly R. Khachadoorian-Elia, M.D., MBA
Chief Resident in Obstetrics & Gynecology
Beth Israel Deaconess Medical Center
Harvard Medical School
Boston, Massachusetts

Obstetrics & Gynecology Contributors

Marisa Dahlman, M.D., MPH
Stephanie Dukhovny, M.D.
Aya Kuribayashi, M.D.
Alice Lo, M.D.
Kavid Nik Udompanyanan, M.D.
Linda C. Yang, M.D.

acknowledgments

Our great thanks to the house staff and faculty from Beth Israel Deaconess, Massachusetts General Hospital, Brigham and Women's, and Children's Hospital in Boston, whose clinical cases, revisions, and suggestions were indispensable to this series.

Thanks to the editors at Lippincott Williams & Wilkins, especially Nancy Hoffmann, who worked overtime on these books.

abbreviations

A-a	alveolar-arterial (oxygen gradient)	ATLS	Advanced Trauma Life Support (protocol)
AAA	abdominal aortic aneurysm	ATN	acute tubular necrosis
ABCs	airway, breathing, circulation	ATPase	adenosine triphosphatase
ABGs	arterial blood gases	ATRA	all-*trans*-retinoic acid
ABPA	allergic bronchopulmonary aspergillosis	AV	arteriovenous, atrioventricular
ABVD	adriamycin, bleomycin, vinblastine, dacarbazine (chemotherapy)	AVPD	avoidant personality disorder
		AXR	abdominal x-ray
		AZT	azidothymidine (zidovudine)
ACE	angiotensin-converting enzyme	BCG	bacille Calmette-Guérin
ACTH	adrenocorticotropic hormone	BE	barium enema
ADA	adenosine deaminase, American Diabetic Association	BP	blood pressure
		BPD	borderline personality disorder
ADH	antidiuretic hormone	BPH	benign prostatic hypertrophy
ADHD	attention-deficit–hyperactivity disorder	BPK	B-cell progenitor kinase
		BPM	beats per minute
AED	automatic external-defibrillator	BUN	blood urea nitrogen
AFP	α-fetoprotein	CAA	cerebral amyloid angiopathy
AI	aortic insufficiency	CABG	coronary artery bypass grafting
AICD	automatic internal cardiac defibrillator	CAD	coronary artery disease
		CALLA	common acute lymphoblastic leukemia antigen
AIDS	acquired immunodeficiency syndrome		
		C-ANCA	cytoplasmic antineutrophil cytoplasmic antibody
ALL	acute lymphocytic leukemia		
ALS	amyotrophic lateral sclerosis	CAO	chronic airway obstruction
ALT	alanine aminotransferase	CAP	community-acquired pneumonia
AML	acute myelogenous leukemia	CBC	complete blood count
AMP	adenosine monophosphate	CBD	common bile duct
ANA	antinuclear antibody	CBT	cognitive behavioral therapy
ANCA	antineutrophil cytoplasmic antibody	CCU	cardiac care unit
		CD	cluster of differentiation
Angio	angiography	CDC	Centers for Disease Control and Prevention
AP	anteroposterior		
aPTT	activated partial thromboplastin time	CEA	carcinoembryonic antigen
		CF	cystic fibrosis
ARDS	adult respiratory distress syndrome	CFTR	cystic fibrosis transmembrane regulator
ARF	acute renal failure	CFU	colony-forming unit
AS	ankylosing spondylitis	CHF	congestive heart failure
ASA	acetylsalicylic acid	CJD	Creutzfeldt–Jakob disease
5-ASA	5-aminosalicylic acid	CK	creatine kinase
ASD	atrial septal defect	CK-MB	creatine kinase, MB fraction
ASO	antistreptolysin O	CLL	chronic lymphocytic leukemia
AST	aspartate aminotransferase	CML	chronic myelogenous leukemia

CMV	cytomegalovirus
CN	cranial nerve
CNS	central nervous system
CO	cardiac output
COPD	chronic obstructive pulmonary disease
CPAP	continuous positive airway pressure
CPK	creatine phosphokinase
CPR	cardiopulmonary resuscitation
CRP	C-reactive protein
CSF	cerebrospinal fluid
CT	computed tomography
CVA	cerebrovascular accident
CXR	chest x-ray
D&C	dilation and curettage
DAF	decay-accelerating factor
DC	direct current
DEXA	dual-energy x-ray absorptiometry
DHEA	dehydroepiandrosterone
DIC	disseminated intravascular coagulation
DIP	distal interphalangeal (joint)
DKA	diabetic ketoacidosis
DL_{CO}	diffusing capacity of carbon monoxide
DM	diabetes mellitus
DMD	Duchenne muscular dystrophy
DNA	deoxyribonucleic acid
DNase	deoxyribonuclease
dsDNA	double-stranded DNA
DTP	diphtheria, tetanus, pertussis (vaccine)
DTRs	deep tendon reflexes
DTs	delirium tremens
DUB	dysfunctional uterine bleeding
DVT	deep venous thrombosis
EBV	Epstein–Barr virus
ECG	electrocardiography
Echo	echocardiography
ECMO	extracorporeal membrane oxygenation
EDTA	ethylenediaminetetraacetic acid
EEG	electroencephalography
EF	ejection fraction
EGD	esophagogastroduodenoscopy
E:I	expiratory-to-inspiratory (ratio)
ELISA	enzyme-linked immunosorbent assay

EM	electron microscopy
EMG	electromyography
ER	emergency room
ERCP	endoscopic retrograde cholangiopancreatography
ESR	erythrocyte sedimentation rate
EtOH	ethanol
FDA	Food and Drug Administration
Fe_{Na}	fractional excretion of sodium
FEV_1	forced expiratory volume in 1 second
FIGO	International Federation of Gynecology and Obstetrics (classification)
FIo_2	fraction of inspired oxygen
FNA	fine-needle aspiration
FRC	functional residual capacity
FSH	follicle-stimulating hormone
FTA	fluorescent treponemal antibody
FTA-ABS	fluorescent treponemal antibody absorption test
5-FU	5-fluorouracil
FVC	forced vital capacity
G6PD	glucose-6-phosphate dehydrogenase
GA	gestational age
GABA	γ-aminobutyric acid
GABHS	group A β-hemolytic streptococci
GAD	generalized anxiety disorder
GBM	glomerular basement membrane
G-CSF	granulocyte–colony-stimulating factor
GERD	gastroesophageal reflux disease
GFR	glomerular filtration rate
GGT	γ-glutamyltransferase
GI	gastrointestinal
GnRH	gonadotropin-releasing hormone
GU	genitourinary
HAV	hepatitis A virus
Hb	hemoglobin
HBcAg	hepatitis B core antigen
HBsAg	hepatitis B surface antigen
HBV	hepatitis B virus
hCG	human chorionic gonadotropin
HCl	hydrogen chloride
HCO_3	bicarbonate
Hct	hematocrit
HCV	hepatitis C virus

HDL	high-density lipoprotein	KOH	potassium hydroxide
HEENT	head, eyes, ears, nose, and throat	KS	Kaposi sarcoma
HELLP	hemolysis, elevated liver enzymes, low platelets (syndrome)	KUB	kidney, ureter, bladder
		LA	left atrium
		LAMB	lentigines, atrial myxoma, blue nevi (syndrome)
HEV	hepatitis E virus	LD	Leishman–Donovan (body)
HGPRT	hypoxanthine-guanine phospho-ribosyltransferase	LDH	lactate dehydrogenase
HHV	human herpesvirus	LDL	low-density lipoprotein
5-HIAA	5-hydroxyindoleacetic acid	LES	lower esophageal sphincter
HIDA	hepato iminodiacetic acid (scan)	LFTs	liver function tests
HIV	human immunodeficiency virus	LH	luteinizing hormone
HLA	human leukocyte antigen	LHRH	luteinizing hormone–releasing hormone
HPF	high-power field		
HPI	history of present illness	I KM	liver–kidney microsomal (antibody)
HPV	human papillomavirus		
HR	heart rate	LMN	lower motor neuron
HRCT	high-resolution computed tomography	LP	lumbar puncture
		L/S	lecithin-to-sphingomyelin (ratio)
HS	hereditary spherocytosis	LSD	lysergic acid diethylamide
HSG	hysterosalpingography	LV	left ventricle, left ventricular
HSV	herpes simplex virus	LVH	left ventricular hypertrophy
HUS	hemolytic–uremic syndrome	Lytes	electrolytes
IABC	intra-aortic balloon counterpulsation	Mammo	mammography
		MAO	monoamine oxidase (inhibitor)
ICA	internal carotid artery	MAP	mean arterial pressure
ICD	implantable cardiac defibrillator	MCA	middle cerebral artery
ICP	intracranial pressure	MCHC	mean corpuscular hemoglobin concentration
ICU	intensive care unit		
ID/CC	identification and chief complaint	MCP	metacarpophalangeal (joint)
IDDM	insulin-dependent diabetes mellitus	MCV	mean corpuscular volume
		MDMA	3,4-methylene-dioxymetham-phetamine ("ecstasy")
IE	infectious endocarditis		
IFA	immunofluorescent antibody	MEN	multiple endocrine neoplasia
Ig	immunoglobulin	MGUS	monoclonal gammopathy of undetermined origin
IL	interleukin		
IM	infectious mononucleosis, intramuscular	MHC	major histocompatibility complex
		MI	myocardial infarction
INH	isoniazid	MIBG	metaiodobenzylguanidine
INR	International Normalized Ratio	MMR	measles, mumps, rubella (vaccine)
123-ISS	iodine-123–labeled somatostatin	MPTP	1-methyl-4-phenyl-tetrahydropy-ridine
IUD	intrauterine device		
IUGR	intrauterine growth retardation	MR	magnetic resonance (imaging)
IV	intravenous		
IVC	inferior vena cava	mRNA	messenger ribonucleic acid
IVIG	intravenous immunoglobulin	MRSA	methicillin-resistant *Staphylococcus aureus*
IVP	intravenous pyelography		
JRA	juvenile rheumatoid arthritis	MS	multiple sclerosis
JVD	jugular venous distention	MTP	metatarsophalangeal (joint)
JVP	jugular venous pressure	MuSK	muscle-specific kinase

MVA	motor vehicle accident	PT	prothrombin time
NADPH	reduced nicotinamide adenine dinucleotide phosphate	PTE	pulmonary thromboembolism
		PTH	parathyroid hormone
NAME	nevi, atrial myxoma, myxoid neurofibroma, ephilides (syndrome)	PTSD	posttraumatic stress disorder
		PTT	partial thromboplastin time
		RA	rheumatoid arthritis, right atrial
NG	nasogastric	RBC	red blood cell
NIDDM	non–insulin-dependent diabetes mellitus	RDW	red-cell distribution width
		REM	rapid eye movement
NMDA	N-methyl-D-aspartate	RF	rheumatoid factor
NPO	nil per os (nothing by mouth)	RhoGAM	Rh immune globulin
NSAID	nonsteroidal anti-inflammatory drug	RNA	ribonucleic acid
		RPR	rapid plasma reagin
Nuc	nuclear medicine	RR	respiratory rate
OCD	obsessive–compulsive disorder	RS	Reed–Sternberg (cell)
OCP	oral contraceptive pill	RSV	respiratory syncytial virus
OCPD	obsessive–compulsive personality disorder	RTA	renal tubular acidosis
		RUQ	right upper quadrant
17-OHP	17-hydroxyprogesterone	RV	residual volume, right ventricle, right ventricular
OPC	organophosphate and carbamate		
OS	opening snap	RVH	right ventricular hypertrophy
OTC	over the counter	SA	sinoatrial
PA	posteroanterior	SAH	subarachnoid hemorrhage
2-PAM	pralidoxime	Sao_2	oxygen saturation in arterial blood
P-ANCA	perinuclear antineutrophil cytoplasmic antibody	SBE	subacute bacterial endocarditis
		SBFT	small bowel follow-through
Pao_2	partial pressure of oxygen	SC	subcutaneous
PAS	periodic acid Schiff	SCC	squamous cell carcinoma
PBS	peripheral blood smear	SIADH	syndrome of inappropriate secretion of antidiuretic hormone
Pco_2	partial pressure of carbon dioxide		
PCOD	polycystic ovary disease	SIDS	sudden infant death syndrome
PCP	phencyclidine	SLE	systemic lupus erythematosus
PCR	polymerase chain reaction	SMA	smooth muscle antibody
PCV	polycythemia vera	SSPE	subacute sclerosing panencephalitis
PDA	patent ductus arteriosus		
PE	physical examination	SSRI	selective serotonin reuptake inhibitor
PEEP	positive end-expiratory pressure		
PET	positron emission tomography	STD	sexually transmitted disease
PFTs	pulmonary function tests	SZPD	schizoid personality disorder
PID	pelvic inflammatory disease	T_3	triiodothyronine
PIP	proximal interphalangeal (joint)	T_4	thyroxine
PKU	phenylketonuria	TAB	therapeutic abortion
PMI	point of maximal impulse	TB	tuberculosis
PMN	polymorphonuclear (leukocyte)	TBSA	total body surface area
PO	per os (by mouth)	TCA	tricyclic antidepressant
Po_2	partial pressure of oxygen	TCD	transcranial Doppler
PPD	purified protein derivative	TD	tardive dyskinesia
PROM	premature rupture of membranes	TENS	transcutaneous electrical nerve stimulation
PRPP	phosphoribosyl pyrophosphate		
PSA	prostate-specific antigen	TFTs	thyroid function tests

THC	*trans*-tetrahydrocannabinol	UGI	upper GI (series)
TIA	transient ischemic attack	UMN	upper motor neuron
TIBC	total iron-binding capacity	URI	upper respiratory infection
TIPS	transjugular intrahepatic	US	ultrasound
	portosystemic shunt	UTI	urinary tract infection
TLC	total lung capacity	UV	ultraviolet
TMJ	temporomandibular joint	VCUG	voiding cystourethrogram
	(syndrome)	VDRL	Venereal Disease Research
TMP-SMX	trimethoprim-sulfamethoxazole		Laboratory
TNF	tumor necrosis factor	VF	ventricular fibrillation
TNM	tumor, node, metastasis (staging)	VIN	vulvar intraepithelial neoplasia
ToRCH	*Toxoplasma,* rubella, CMV,	VLDL	very low density lipoprotein
	herpes zoster	VMA	vanillylmandelic acid
tPA	tissue plasminogen activator	V/Q	ventilation-perfusion (ratio)
TPO	thyroid peroxidase	VS	vital signs
TRAP	tartrate-resistant acid	VSD	ventricular septal defect
	phosphatase	VT	ventricular tachycardia
TRH	thyrotropin-releasing hormone	vWF	von Willebrand factor
TSH	thyroid-stimulating hormone	VZIG	varicella-zoster immune
TSS	toxic shock syndrome		globulin
TSST	toxic shock syndrome toxin	VZV	varicella-zoster virus
TTP	thrombotic thrombocytopenic	WAGR	Wilms tumor, aniridia, ambigu-
	purpura		ous genitalia, mental retardation
TUBD	transurethral balloon dilatation		(syndrome)
TUIP	transurethral incision of the	WBC	white blood cell
	prostate	WG	Wegener granulomatosis
TURP	transurethral resection of the	WPW	Wolff–Parkinson White
	prostate		(syndrome)
UA	urinalysis	XR	x-ray

Underground Clinical Vignettes

Obstetrics and Gynecology

FOURTH EDITION

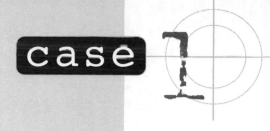

ID/CC A 28-year-old recently married woman complains of an **offensive vaginal discharge**.

HPI She states that the discharge is **thin, white, and foul-smelling**. She reports no vulvar pruritus or soreness. No dysuria or dyspareunia.

PE VS: no fever. PE: speculum examination reveals homogenous, grayish-white, watery discharge coating the vaginal walls. There is a **"fishy" odor** (due to volatile amines) **upon mixing with 10% KOH** (POSITIVE "WHIFF" TEST).

Micro Pathology Vaginal **pH >4.5**; saline smear reveals characteristic **"clue cells"** (squamous epithelial cells with stippled borders due to adherent bacteria). UA: normal.

case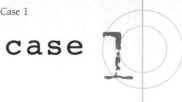

Bacterial Vaginosis

Pathogenesis

Bacterial vaginosis occurs when normal *Lactobacillus* in the vagina is **replaced by high concentrations of anaerobic bacteria,** including *Bacteroides, Peptostreptococcus,* and *Mobiluncus* species. *Gardnerella vaginalis,* now recognized as normal vaginal flora, is found in increased concentrations in 90% of cases. Risk factors include multiple sexual partners, early age of first coitus, douching, smoking, and use of intrauterine device. Bacterial vaginosis increases the risks of pelvic inflammatory disease, chorioamnionitis, preterm labor, premature rupture of membranes, and postpartum endometritis.

Management

All symptomatic women should be treated. Treat with a 7-day course of **metronidazole.** Clindamycin is also effective. Treatment can be offered during pregnancy (metronidazole is contraindicated during the first trimester; topical clindamycin is contraindicated during the third trimester because of the risk of premature delivery). Treatment of sexual partners is not indicated. Women with recurrent or persistent bacterial vaginosis should be screened for STDs.

Breakout Point

- Patients taking metronidazole should not drink alcohol, as it leads to a disulfiram-like reaction.
- Bacterial vaginosis is the most common cause of vaginitis in women of childbearing age.

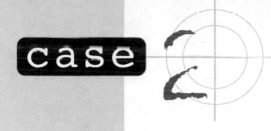

case 2

ID/CC A 27-year-old woman complains of **painful, unilateral vulvar swelling.**

HPI She reports a 3-day history of a swelling in her left labia that has increased in size and pain. She has **difficulty walking and sitting** because of the discomfort. She has also been experiencing **dyspareunia** (painful intercourse). She denies fevers or chills.

PE VS: afebrile. Inspection of the vulvar region reveals **swelling of the left labia majorum. A tender 4-cm mass** is palpable at the **4-o'clock position.** No erythema or warmth is observed.

Micro Pathology *Chlamydia* and gonococcal cultures negative. Urinalysis normal.

case 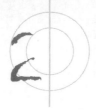 2

Bartholin Cyst

Pathogenesis

Bartholin glands are paired glandular structures located at the **4-o'clock and 8-o'clock positions on the posterolateral aspect of the vestibule.** They are each drained by a single duct that **exits just external to the hymenal ring.** Cyst development occurs with blockage of the duct and accumulation of mucinous material. Infection of a Bartholin gland cyst can result in abscess formation that can be characterized by fever and redness or warmth in the gland area.

Management

Asymptomatic cysts do not require treatment in pre-menopausal women. Conservative management with warm compresses and sitz baths can help alleviate symptoms. Other options, of increasing invasiveness, include incision and drainage, incision and drainage with Word catheter placement, marsupialization of the cyst, or cyst excision. **The most common intervention is incision and drainage with Word catheter placement,** indicated for acute cyst pain. The bulb of the catheter is inflated and should remain for at least 2 to 4 weeks to promote formation of an epithelialized tract. Broad-spectrum antibiotics are only recommended in cases of abscess formation. If patient experiences recurrent Bartholin cyst formation, then more invasive options should be considered.

Complications

Prognosis for Bartholin gland cysts is typically good following appropriate treatment, without significant long-term effects. Bartholin gland abscesses can lead to serious infectious complications and, rarely, sepsis.

Breakout Point

- Rule out malignancy in postmenopausal women with tissue biopsy.
- Diabetes mellitus makes infection more likely.
- Test for concomitant gonococcal and *Chlamydia* infections.
- Consider marsupialization or excision procedures in recurrent cases.
- Antibiotics should only be prescribed if there are signs or symptoms of infection.

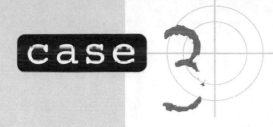

case 3

ID/CC A 21-year-old college student presents to the student health clinic with **dysuria**.

HPI Patient reports 2 to 3 days of having a **burning pain at the labia** as the urine passes. She denies suprapubic discomfort, but has had **vaginal itching** for the preceding week with **thick white vaginal discharge**. There is no urinary frequency or urgency, or dyspareunia. She recently completed a course of a cephalosporin **antibiotic** for a skin infection.

PE VS: normal. Nontender abdomen. Speculum examination reveals erythematous, edematous labial and vaginal mucosa. **A white, adherent, "cottage cheese"-like discharge** is present in the vaginal vault. Cervix is unremarkable.

Micro Pathology Vaginal pH is **<4.5**. UA: negative. Wet mount with KOH reveals **pseudohyphae with buds**.

■ TABLE 3-1 VAGINAL DISCHARGE

	Physiologic	*Candida*	Bacterial Vaginosis	*Trichomonas*	Atrophic
Symptoms	None	Pruritus, burning	± Pruritus, burning	± Pruritus	± Vulvar, vaginal dryness
Malodor	None	Yeast smell	Fishy or musty	Variable	Variable
Increased mucosal erythema	None	Yes	±	Yes	±
Consistency	Floccular	Thick, curd-like	Thin, creamy	Copious, trothy	Mucoid, blood tinge
pH	3.8–4.5	3.5–4.5	5.0–6.0	6.0–7.0	As high as 7.0
Wet smear	Rare WBCs, large gram-positive rods, squamous epithelial cells	Budding filaments, spores, pseudohyphae	Clue cells	Copious WBCs, trichomonads	Copious WBCs, parabasal and intermediate cells, paucity of superficial cells
Potassium Hydroxide preparation		Budding filaments, spores, pseudohyphae	Fishy odor, musty odor	—	—
Treatment of choice	None	Imidazole or triazole derivative	Metronidazole or clindamycin	Metronidazole	Estrogen cream

WBCs, white blood cells.

5

case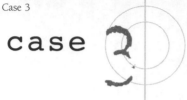

Candidal Vaginitis

Pathogenesis

Approximately 80% to 95% of cases of fungal vaginitis are caused by *Candida albicans*. *Candida* is a normal colonizer in approximately 25% of women. Symptomatic infection typically occurs when vaginal flora are altered by **hormonal factors** (including oral contraception and pregnancy), **depressed cellular immunity**, or **antibiotics. Diabetes** is also a risk factor.

Management

Many **azole preparations** are available over the counter (butoconazole, clotrimazole, miconazole, tioconazole, terconazole), in creams or vaginal suppositories. A **single oral dose of fluconazole** is also effective and may be preferred by patients for its ease of use, although it can adversely affect liver function. Pregnant women should be treated with a topical regimen. Treatment of sexual partners is not indicated.

Breakout Point

- In patients who have recurrent candidal vaginitis, screen for diabetes and perform a culture for identification and sensitivities of the pathogen.
- Sensitivity of wet mount for *Candida* is about 65%. If clinical picture is strongly suggestive for candidiasis but wet mount is negative, perform a culture.
- Asymptomatic women and sexual partners of symptomatic patients do not need to be treated.

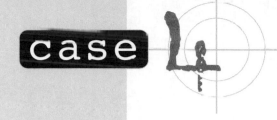

case 4

ID/CC An 18-year-old female college student presents for her annual examination.

HPI The patient is sexually active, has had five partners in the last year, and is on oral contraceptive pills. She reports mildly increased yellow vaginal discharge over the past month. She denies dysuria.

PE VS: normal. Abdomen is nontender. Speculum examination reveals a **friable cervix** with a visible **ectropion** (eversion of the cervix) and yellowish **purulent discharge** exuding from the os. Bimanual examination is unremarkable.

Labs CBC normal.

Micro Pathology **Gram stain** from cervical discharge was obtained, which was read as negative. **The nucleic acid amplification tests (NAAT)** return positive for *Chlamydia*, negative for gonorrhea.

■ TABLE 4-1 TREATMENT REGIMENS FOR GONORRHEA AND *CHLAMYDIA*

Gonorrhea
Recommended loading dose regimen (choice of one plus treatment for *Chlamydia*)
    Ceftriaxone (Rocephin), 125 mg IM
    Cefixime (Suprax), 400 mg PO
    Ciprofloxacin (Cipro), 500 mg PO
    Ofloxacin (Floxin), 400 mg PO
    Levofloxacin (Levaquin) 250 mg PO
Alternative regimen (choice of one)
    Spectinomycin (Trobicin), 2 g IM
    Ceftizoxime (Cefizox), 500 mg IM; cefotaxime (Claforan), 500 mg IM; or cefoxitin (Mefoxin), 1 g IM with probenecid
    Norfloxacin (Noroxin), 800 mg PO or gatifloxacin (Tequin) 400 mg PO; all in a single dose

Chlamydia
Follow-up regimen to treat *Chlamydia* (choice of one)
    Azithromycin (Zithromax), 1 g PO, in a single dose, *or* doxycycline, 100 mg PO, bid for 7 days
Alternative regimen (choice of one)
    Ofloxacin, 300 mg PO bid for 7 days
    Erythromycin (see "Pregnant patients," below)
    Levofloxacin 500 mg PO for 7 days
Pregnant patients (choice of one)
    Preferred regimen
        Erythromycin base 500 mg PO qid for 7 days, *or*
        Amoxicillin 500 mg PO tid for 7 days, *or*
        Azithromycin,
        Erythromycin base, 250 mg PO qid for 14 days; *or*
        Azithromycin
    Alternative regimen
        Erythromycin ethylsuccinate, 800 mg PO qid or 400 mg PO qid for 14 days

case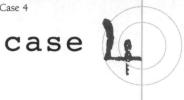

Cervicitis

Pathogenesis

Cervicitis is frequently asymptomatic, or may be noted on PE when the cervix is extremely friable. *Neisseria gonorrhoeae* or *Chlamydia trachomatis* is isolated in approximately 50% of patients with purulent cervical discharge. *Chlamydia* cervicitis is a sexually transmitted disease, and is most likely to occur in adolescents or young adults. The causative organism, *C. trachomatis*, is a small gram-negative bacterium; it is an obligate intracellular parasite. Risk factors for *Chlamydia* cervicitis include **multiple sex partners, unprotected sex,** history of **other sexually transmitted disease,** and **cervical ectopy.**

Management

All patients should be treated for presumed *C. trachomatis* infection (because it is more often missed on testing), even if the organism is not isolated. If *N. gonorrhoeae* is isolated, patients should receive treatment for both organisms. **Azithromycin or doxycycline** is used to treat *Chlamydia*; a third-generation cephalosporin (e.g., **ceftriaxone) or fluoroquinolone is** used for gonorrhea. Test to ascertain cure should be performed in 3 months.

Complications

In untreated cervicitis, the infection may ascend and cause pelvic inflammatory disease or tubo-ovarian abscess. Long-term complications can include intra-abdominal adhesions, hydrosalpinx, and infertility.

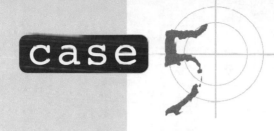

case 5

ID/CC A 22-year-old woman presents after recently noticing two **pruritic "bumps"** on her **vulva and perineum.**

HPI The lesions also cause a "**burning**" sensation. She denies any vaginal discharge, dysuria, or hematuria She is **sexually active** with **multiple partners** and does not use any form of birth control.

PE PE: Soft, pink, pedunculated growths 5 to 7 mm in diameter.

Labs CBC: normal. RPR: nonreactive.

Gross Pathology **Diagnostic biopsy** reveals papillomatous elongation and parakeratosis with cytoplasmic vacuolization (**koilocytes**).

Micro Pathology Cultures for gonorrhea and *Chlamydia* negative. Tzanck smear negative for HSV. Vaginal wet mount and KOH negative.

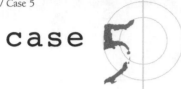

case

Condylomata Acuminata

Pathogenesis

There are more than 70 different subtypes **of human papillomavirus,** which are double-stranded DNA viruses. Condylomata acuminata and low-grade intraepithelial neoplasia are most frequently associated with **subtypes 6 and 11,** which do not integrate into the host genome. **Subtypes 16 and 18** are associated with squamous carcinoma of the cervix, vulva, vagina, anus, penis, and bladder. The virus is transmitted by vaginal and anal **intercourse.** Risk factors include **immunosuppression, multiple sexual partners, HIV, and other forms of sexually transmitted diseases**. Circumcised men are less likely to be infected with HPV then uncircumcised men.

Epidemiology

HPV is the most common sexually transmitted virus.

Management

Obtain **Pap smear** and perform a thorough PE to document extent of lesions. Five-percent acetic acid turns the lesion white and may facilitate diagnosis. Biopsy is recommended when the diagnosis is uncertain from visual inspection, or when carcinoma is suspected, especially for ulcerated lesions or if treatments below are ineffective. Asymptomatic lesions may be observed, and spontaneous resolution may occur in 20% of cases. Bothersome symptoms (pruritis, bleeding, burning) are indications for treatment. Small warts may be treated with local application of 25% **podophyllin** (contraindicated during pregnancy, and not to be used on mucosal surfaces because it results in chemical burns), **podophyllotoxin** (the active compound of podophyllin), **trichloroacetic acid** (preferred treatment for pregnant women), **imiquimod,** topical 5-FU or freezing with **liquid nitrogen** (another safe option for pregnant women). Other options include **laser** removal, **electrocautery,** intralesional **interferon,** or **surgical removal** (large lesions). Treatment does not usually eradicate HPV from the anogenital area, so transmission to sexual partners is still possible. Recurrence rates may be up to 70% after treatment.

Complications

Cervical lesions require monitoring via routine Pap smears and/or colposcopy for **cervical neoplasia.**

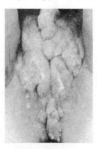

Figure 5-1. Vulvar condylomata acuminata lesions.

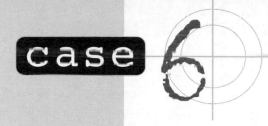

ID/CC A 32-year-old G2P2 presents **desiring a new form of contraception.**

HPI She delivered 6 weeks ago and would like long-term contraception. She previously was on birth control pills but acknowledges that it has been difficult to remember to take her daily dose. She and her husband are uncertain of their desire for future children and do not like the feel of condoms. She has a history of depression but no other history of illness or disease (gonorrhea or *Chlamydia*). She has regular periods lasting 4 to 5 days with light flow.

PE Afebrile, stable vital signs. Uterus is anteverted and normal in size.

case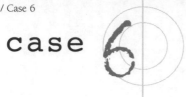

Contraception

Pathogenesis Women who desire long-term contraception but do not like the feel of (or are allergic to) condoms, or experience negative side-effects of oral contraceptive pills, may be offered one of two currently available intrauterine devices: copper T-380A intrauterine device (ParaGard) or the levonorgestrel-releasing intrauterine system.

Management Gonorrhea and *Chlamydia* testing, followed by IUD placement.

Complications Infection, uterine perforation, possible future pregnancy, possible ectopic pregnancy.

Breakout Point

> • Contraception is lifestyle-dependent, because effectiveness is directly affected by patient compliance.
> • Correct use and actual use rates can vary widely.
> • For patient considering sterilization, male sterilization should also be presented as an option during counseling.

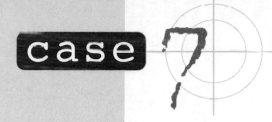

ID/CC A 17-year-old G0 is seen with complaints of **irregular, prolonged, and excessive menstrual bleeding.**

HPI Patient reports periods lasting 8 to 12 days, sometimes requiring her to change her pads every 1/2 hour. Her menarche was at age 12, and her periods have always been somewhat irregular. Over the last 6 months, her periods have become more irregular, occurring anytime between 14 and 45 days. She denies breast tenderness, pelvic pain, or vaginal discharge, and has never been sexually active. No history of easy bruisability.

PE VS: normal. PE: obese young woman, with minimal acne and no abnormal hair growth. No thyroid enlargement noted. Pelvic examination reveals no lesions on the vulva, vagina, or cervix. A normal-sized uterus is noted, with no palpable adnexa or other masses. There is no cervical motion tenderness.

Labs CBC: hypochromic, microcytic anemia; Hct 28. Lytes: normal. PT/PTT: normal. UA: normal. TSH, FSH, and prolactin normal; pregnancy test negative.

Imaging Pelvic ultrasound reveals a normal anteverted uterus with no uterine masses and a normal endometrium, and normal ovaries bilaterally.

■ TABLE 7-1 CAUSES OF DYSFUNCTIONAL UTERINE BLEEDING

Type of Bleed	Clinical Examples
Estrogen withdrawal	Bleeding after discontinuation or decrease in estrogen (after oophorectomy or pelvic radiation; midcycle bleeding; HRT tapering).
Estrogen breakthrough	Breakdown in endometrial tissue that was stimulated by high estrogen levels or sustained exposure to estrogen (obesity, PCOS). Chronic low-dose estrogen can also cause intermittent spotting.
Progesterone withdrawal	Discontinuation of progesterone (removal of corpus luteum, progesterone withdrawal trial during infertility workup). Requires some endometrial proliferation by estrogen.
Progesterone breakthrough	Spotting after continuous progesterone therapy in the absence of sufficient estrogen (Depo-Provera and long-term OCPs).

13

case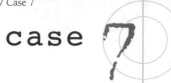

Dysfunctional Uterine Bleeding

Pathogenesis

Dysfunctional uterine bleeding (DUB) can be **anovulatory (more common)** or **ovulatory**. In anovulatory DUB, no corpus luteum develops and progesterone is absent. Unopposed estrogen results in proliferation, necrosis, and random, asynchronous shedding of the endometrium, which causes irregular bleeding. In ovulatory DUB, the corpus luteum develops but does not secrete enough progesterone to stabilize the endometrium, also known as luteal phase defect.

Epidemiology

The two peaks of incidence of abnormal uterine bleeding are puberty and the perimenopausal years (more common). Infrequent menorrhagia is also associated with **polycystic ovary syndrome**, which is a syndrome of **irregular menses, obesity, hirsutism/acne, and insulin resistance.**

Management

Irregular menses can be caused by **thyroid disease, hyperprolactinemia,** or **decreased ovarian reserve** (especially in the perimenopausal population). **TSH** and **prolactin** levels should be checked in all patients, with **FSH** checked for women who are having menopausal symptoms such as hot flashes. A **pregnancy test** and **Pap smear** should also be done to eliminate pregnancy or cervical cancer as a source. Imaging, by **pelvic ultrasound** or saline sonohystogram, is helpful for identifying any structural cause (fibroids or endometrial polyps), which can be corrected via hysteroscopy. For women at high risk for **endometrial carcinoma** (e.g., increased estrogen exposure), endometrial biopsy and hysteroscopy can be helpful in ruling out carcinoma. After underlying pathologic conditions have been ruled out, **NSAIDs, OCPs, or cyclical progestogens may be given to regulate menstruation and prevent excessive bleeding on a long-term basis.** D&C may be indicated for protracted or refractory bleeding. For women who have completed childbearing, endometrial ablation and uterine artery embolization are also available. Definitive surgical treatment is hysterectomy. Iron supplementation recommended for iron-deficiency anemia.

Complications

Anemia; endometrial intraepithelial lesion (formerly known as endometrial hyperplasia) with risk of carcinoma.

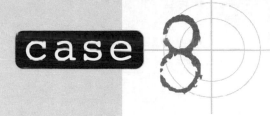
ID/CC A 17-year-old G0 girl presents with **cyclic lower abdominal cramping** occurring during menses.

HPI She states that her symptoms **began shortly after menarche.** She frequently misses school because of the severity of the pain. She often experiences **bloating and back pain** during menstruation. Her flow is not heavy, and she changes her pad 3 or 4 times a day during her periods, which last 5 days. She is sexually active.

PE VS: normal. Pelvic examination demonstrates normal external female genitalia and an anteverted, mobile uterus. **No cul-de-sac nodularity** or adnexal masses are appreciated.

Labs Serum β-hCG: <5 mIU/mL.

Imaging Pelvic ultrasound normal.

Micro Pathology Gonococcal and *Chlamydia* cultures negative.

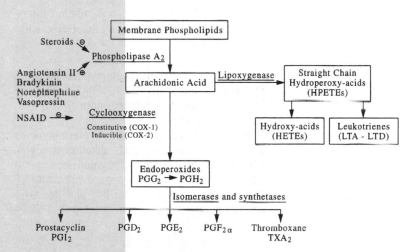

Figure 8-1. Arachidonic acid pathway and prostaglandin production. (NSAID, nonsteroidal anti-inflammatory drug; PG, prostaglandin.) Cramping pain is associated with excess prostaglandin in production.

case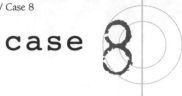

Dysmenorrhea

Pathogenesis

Dysmenorrhea is classified as either primary or secondary. Primary dysmenorrhea is associated with ovulatory cycles and is more prevalent in **adolescents**. This condition is associated with **excess prostaglandin production** (prostaglandin $F_{2\alpha}$). Secondary dysmenorrhea is defined as menstrual pain related to underlying pelvic pathology such as endometriosis, pelvic inflammatory disease, or other structural lesions.

Management

Nonsteroidal anti-inflammatory drugs (NSAIDs) are effective for the treatment of primary dysmenorrhea in 80% of patients. In patients without contraindications and who desire contraception, **hormonal contraceptives** can also be used and may achieve symptomatic relief in over 90% of patients. Failure to respond to these initial therapies warrants further investigation for causes of secondary dysmenorrhea.

Complications

Primary dysmenorrhea may lead to significant interference with daily activities, but is not associated with major complications.

Breakout Point

- Dysmenorrhea is the most common menstrual problem in adolescents.
- Pelvic examination is typically normal in primary dysmenorrhea.
- NSAIDs block the conversion of arachidonic acid to prostaglandins and leukotrienes via inhibition of the enzyme cyclooxygenase.
- Hormonal contraception is a good option for women who have dysmenorrhea and desire contraception.

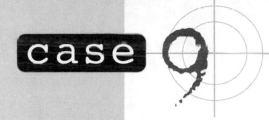

ID/CC	A 27-year-old woman presents with **pelvic pain that occurs with menses.**
HPI	There is an **increase in the quantity and frequency of her menstrual periods** (HYPERPOLYMENORRHEA) and frequent spotting. She has also experienced progressively worsening **dysmenorrhea** and **pain during coitus** (DYSPAREUNIA). She has been unsuccessfully trying to get pregnant for 12 months **(infertility).**
PE	VS: mild hypotension (BP 100/60); no fever. PE: umbilical area shows 3-mm **hyperpigmented, raised, nontender nodule** (extrapelvic endometrial implant); pelvic examination reveals **fixed, retroverted uterus** with **tender nodularity in uterosacral ligament;** cervix normal; **diagnostic laparoscopy** reveals multiple rust-colored ("POWDER BURN") endometrial implants in ovaries, round and broad ligaments, tubes, and cul-de-sac with adhesions.
Labs	CBC/Lytes: normal. TFTs: normal. Infertility panel normal in patient and spouse.
Imaging	US, abdomen: cystic masses in both ovaries.
Gross Pathology	Biopsies of endometrial implants reveal **stroma and glands** identical to endometrium.
Micro Pathology	UA: normal.

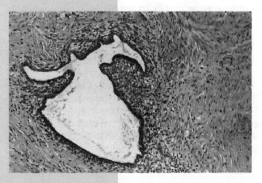

Figure 9-1. Island of ectopic endometrial gland and stroma within the wall of the urinary bladder.

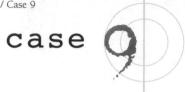

case

Endometriosis

Pathogenesis

Endometriosis is **abnormal implantation of endometrial tissue** outside the uterine cavity, leading to infertility, dyspareunia, and dysmenorrhea. Three theories on the pathogenesis of endometriosis include the **Halban theory** (endometrial tissue spreads via lymphatic channels), **retrograde menstruation** (endometrial tissue spreads via fallopian tubes), and **metaplastic transformation** (multipotent cells become functional endometrial tissue). **Family history** of the disease, **retrograde menstruation**, and a history of **prolonged hyperpolymenorrhea** have all been associated with an increased risk of developing symptomatic endometriosis. Endometriomas (CHOCOLATE CYSTS) may also be seen, which look like bilateral **ovarian** cystic masses (containing fluid or blood). The diagnosis can be made only by visual inspection of the abdomen (laparoscopy or laparotomy).

Epidemiology

Mean age of presentation is 27, but incidence is not linked to age or race. Approximately 10% of women will develop endometriosis.

Management

Diagnostic laparoscopy should be done in any woman suspected to have endometriosis. The first line of treatment is usually NSAIDs in conjunction with **OCPs** are given to suppress stimulation and growth of endometrial implants. More aggressive endometriosis may be managed with Depo-Provera (IM progesterone), Lupron (a GnRH analog), or Danazol (an androgen derivative). **Surgical measures** include laparoscopic coagulation, laser ablation of lesions, or open surgery with removal of lesions and freeing of adhesions; these measures may improve fertility. In cases involving chronic pain refractory to medical treatment or when childbearing is complete, a **total hysterectomy with bilateral salpingo-oophorectomy** may be indicated.

Complications

Disabling pain, infertility refractory to treatment, and recurrent disease when an ovary is preserved after hysterectomy. Endometriosis is a risk factor for ovarian cancer development.

Breakout Point

- Ectopic endometrial implants are most often found in the pelvis, but can be *anywhere* in the body.
- CA-125 may be elevated for women with endometriosis, but does not mean they have ovarian cancer.
- Menopause leads to decreased ovarian hormonal levels, and thus cessation of endometriosis symptoms.

case 10

ID/CC A 19-year-old college student presents to a walk-in clinic with **vaginal discharge** and **intermittent spotting between menses.**

HPI Patient has noted spotting since her spontaneous abortion 2 months prior. Spotting most often occurs **after intercourse** and is **scant.** One month ago she noted an increase in odorless **vaginal discharge**, leading her to self-medicate for a yeast infection, with no change in symptoms. She is monogamous with a single male partner for several years. Her last menstrual period was 2 weeks ago, which was heavier than usual.

PE VS: normal. Nontender abdomen. Speculum examination reveals normal urethra and vaginal mucosa. The cervix is inflamed and **bleeds easily** when swabbed. There is **mucopurulent cervical discharge** at the os. Bartholin and Skene glands are normal. Bimanual examination is unremarkable.

Labs CBC: normal.

Micro Pathology **Urinalysis** and wet mount are normal. **Gram stain** from cervical discharge was obtained, which was read as negative. **The nucleic acid amplification tests (NAAT)** return positive for gonorrhea, negative for *Chlamydia.*

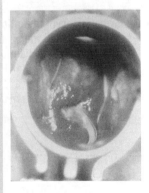

Figure 10-1. Mucopurulent discharge at the cervical os.

19

case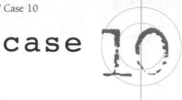

Gonorrhea

Pathogenesis

Neisseria gonorrhoeae is a **gram-negative aerobic diplococcus** with a predilection for mucosal surfaces. The most common primary site of infection is endocervical, although concurrent pharyngeal and anorectal involvement is not uncommon. Acquisition is though mucosal sexual contact with an infected partner.

Management

Treat for both gonorrhea (ceftriaxone, or fluoroquinolones such as ciprofloxacin or levofloxacin) and *Chlamydia* (doxycycline or azithromycin), because *Chlamydia* is more often missed on testing than is gonorrhea. Pregnant women should avoid fluoroquinolones and tetracyclines, and should be treated with ceftriaxone and azithromycin instead. Sexual partners should be identified and treated. Both should abstain from sex until treatment is complete.

Complications

Pelvic inflammatory disease (10%–20% of infected women) potentially leading to infertility. Fitz–Hugh–Curtis syndrome, or perihepatitis, with right upper quadrant pain/tenderness and abnormal LFTs. Ophthalmia neonatorum if mother is infected during delivery. Disseminated gonococcal infection (1%–3% incidence) with septic arthritis/osteomyelitis, endocarditis, and meningitis may also occur.

Breakout Point

- Gonorrhea is **asymptomatic in 50% to 80% of women** (but asymptomatic in only 10% of men).
- Gold standard for diagnosis is culture on Thayer-Martin medium or PCR.
- Women who test positive for gonorrhea should also be treated for *Chlamydia*.

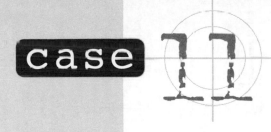

case 11

ID/CC	A 32-year-old G2P0010 is referred to a clinic for **inability to conceive.**
HPI	The patient was married 1 year ago, has not used any form of contraception, and has had unprotected sexual intercourse at least twice a week. She had a therapeutic abortion 7 years ago, complicated by a pelvic infection, and notes irregular and painful menses since then. She denies any other medical or surgical history. Neither she nor her husband has ever had children.
PE	VS: normal. PE: normal neurologic examination with full visual fields; no thyromegaly; normal breast examination; abdomen soft and nontender; pelvic examination reveals uterus of normal size with no masses and no cervical motion tenderness; adnexa not palpable; vagina and cervix appear normal.
Labs	CBC/Lytes/UA: normal. TFTs, FSH normal; cortisol, prolactin, testosterone, and DHEA levels normal.
Imaging	Pelvic US: normal uterus with an irregular endometrial stripe but no adnexal masses. HSG: two intrauterine synechiae in the midbody of the endometrial cavity and patent fallopian tubes.

▓ **TABLE 11-1 CAUSES OF INFERTILITY AND THEIR APPROXIMATE FREQUENCIES**

Main Causes

Sperm defects or dysfunction, 30% (including spermatogenic failure [complete or virtually complete failure leading to azoospermia] in 1%–2%, seminal sperm antibodies in 5%, and varicocele in 1%–2%)
Ovulation failure (amenorrhea or oligomenorrhea), 25% (including primary ovarian failure in 1%–2%)
Tubal infective damage, 20%
Unexplained infertility, 25%

Other Causes

Endometriosis (causing tubal or ovarian structural damage), 5%
Coital failure or infrequency, 5%
Cervical mucus defects or dysfunction, 3%
Uterine abnormalities (e.g., fibroids), rare as a true cause
Genital tuberculosis, rare in developed countries
General debilitating illnesses, rare

case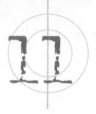

Infertility

Pathogenesis

Infertility is the inability to conceive in 1 year of regular sexual intercourse without contraception. The most common causes of infertility are **lack of normal spermatogenesis, lack of ovulatory cycles,** and **anatomic defects of the female genitalia.** Causes of male infertility include mumps orchitis with atrophy, antisperm antibodies, Klinefelter syndrome, retrograde ejaculation, testicular varicocele, hypogonadotropic hypogonadism, and Sertoli-cell-only syndrome. Female anatomic abnormalities that can cause infertility include congenital defects; acquired defects such as **Asherman syndrome,** which is intrauterine adhesion (SYNECHIAE) formation due to previous vigorous curettage of the uterus or infections such as tuberculosis; PID, which produces adhesions that may obstruct the fallopian tubes; leiomyomata; and endometriosis.

Epidemiology

Infertility affects 15% of couples in the reproductive age group. Male factor is the attributed cause in approximately 25% of cases. In 30% of cases, infertility is unexplained.

Management

Occurrence of ovulation should be established in any infertility workup. Ovulation may be ascertained via **measurement of luteal-phase progesterone levels** or following **basal body temperature.** Women with biphasic temperature curves are likely ovulatory, with a peak temperature seen in consonance with the rise in progesterone following LH surge. **Hysterosalpingography** can show irregularities in the endometrial cavity and patency of the fallopian tubes. **Laparoscopy** is very helpful in diagnosing and treating endometriosis and adhesion formation. **Male-factor infertility** should also be evaluated. More than 75% of infertile couples eventually conceive with treatment. Treatment varies according to the cause and ranges from **induction of ovulation with clomiphene or gonadotropins** to surgical correction of anatomic abnormalities, in vitro fertilization, and intrauterine insemination.

Complications

With assisted reproductive technology, multiple-gestation pregnancies and premature delivery.

Breakout Point

- Infertility is the inability to conceive within 1 year of intercourse without contraception.
- Cause of infertility is equal between male and female factors, but 30% remains idiopathic.
- Workup of infertility includes a semen analysis of the male partner as well as evaluating ovulation and possible structural defects in the female partner.

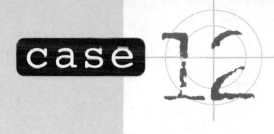
ID/CC A 58-year-old woman complains of **shortness of breath** and **abdominal distention.**

HPI She has had worsening shortness of breath over several days, and increasing abdominal distention over several months. She notes some weight loss but no changes in eating habits or bowel movements.

PE VS: tachypneic (respiratory rate 24). Oxygen saturation is 93% on room air. Examination is significant for a thin woman with increased work of breathing. **Decreased breath sounds in right lung.** Abdomen is nontender but markedly distended, with **palpable fluid wave.** Pelvic examination reveals a large **right adnexal mass.**

Labs CBC normal. Cytology of the ascitic fluid yields no malignant cells. CA-125 level is elevated.

Imaging CXR confirms large right pleural effusion. CT, abdomen: large amount of ascites as well as a 10-cm solid right ovarian mass.

Gross Pathology Pathology of the mass during surgery is consistent with a fibroma.

case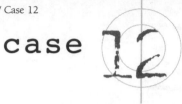

Meigs Syndrome

Pathogenesis

Meigs syndrome is a **triad of ascites, pleural effusion, and ovarian fibroma.** The cause of ascites and pleural effusion development is unclear, but thought to possibly be due to increased secretion of VEGF.

Management

Paracentesis and thoracentesis can be done for symptomatic relief. A unilateral salpingo-oophorectomy is recommended for definitive treatment.

Complications

The clinical presentation is the same as in ovarian cancer. Any suspicion of malignancy requires staging laparotomy with pelvic and periaortic lymph node sampling, as well as total abdominal hysterectomy, bilateral salpingo-oophorectomy in women who are not concerned with fertility.

Breakout Point

- Meigs syndrome is a triad of ascites, pleural effusion, and ovarian fibroma.
- Pseudo–Meigs syndrome is the same triad but with a benign nonfibroma mass.
- Ovarian cancer can present with similar clinical picture and lab results.
- CA-125 is neither a screening nor definitive test for ovarian cancer, and can be elevated in many benign diseases.
- Women with Meigs syndrome must have an endometrial biopsy to rule out concurrent endometrial cancer.

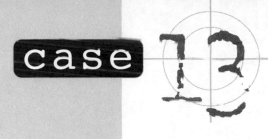

case 13

ID/CC   A **51-year-old** woman complains of **hot flashes, night sweats, emotional lability,** depression, sleep disturbance, and inability to concentrate.

HPI   She also notes **decreased libido, painful coitus** (DYSPAREUNIA) due to decreased vaginal lubrication, and **painful micturition** (DYSURIA). Her last menstrual period was 13 months ago.

PE   Gynecologic examination reveals **atrophic vaginitis.**

Labs   Labs are rarely checked for this condition, but can find **elevated FSH and LH levels; cholesterol and triglycerides increased** in relation to prior levels (decreased HDL and increased LDL and VLDL).

Imaging   CXR, spine: decreased bone density. DEXA: **osteoporosis.**

case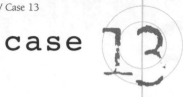

Menopause

Pathogenesis

Menopause is the **cessation of menstrual periods due to a decline in estrogen and progesterone production from the ovaries.** The number of oocytes capable of responding to LH and FSH decreases, and anovulation becomes more frequent. **Decreased estrogen production,** via the feedback loop, leads to **increased LH and FSH** levels, which causes the vasomotor symptoms of menopause. The peripheral conversion of adrenal androstenedione to estrogen becomes the principal source of estrogen after menopause.

Management

Hormonal replacement therapy (HRT) should consist of estrogen-progesterone therapy for women in whom the uterus is still present; unopposed estrogen therapy can be given in women who have had a hysterectomy (**unopposed estrogen therapy increases the risk of endometrial cancer** by inducing atypical adenomatous hyperplasia). Hormone replacement should be instituted at the lowest possible doses and for the shortest period of time. Treatment benefits include **decreased risk for osteoporosis and cardiovascular disease;** side effects include **increased risk of DVT,** cholestatic hepatic dysfunction, and **estrogen-dependent cancers (breast, ovary). Calcium supplementation** and weight-bearing exercises should be prescribed for prevention of osteoporosis.

Breakout Point

- Mean age is 51 years old.
- "Early menopause" is defined by menopause between ages 40 and 45. "Premature ovarian failure" is defined by reaching menopause before age 40.

■ TABLE 13-1 STAGES OF MENOPAUSAL TRANSITION

Stage	Description
Premenopause	Reproductive years
Perimenopause	Cycles of variable length, or skipped cycles. May have hot flashes starting in this stage. Women are in this stage until menopause is reached.
Menopause	Defined by 12 months of amenorrhea after the last menstrual period
Postmenopause	Time after menopause is reached until death

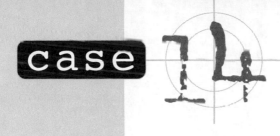

ID/CC   A 23-year-old woman presents to the emergency room with **lower abdominal pain.**

HPI   Patient states that the pain began about 3 days ago. The pain is **bilateral**, and she reports a **dull, constant pressure** in the pelvis. She denies nausea/vomiting/ diarrhea, or dysuria. She has been using an **intrauterine device** since becoming sexually active with her **new partner.** Her **last menstrual period was 1 week ago.**

PE   VS: temperature 100.5°F, HR 100. On abdominal examination, there is **tenderness to palpation in bilateral lower quadrants.** Speculum examination reveals a **mucopurulent cervical discharge** with a **friable cervix.** The patient is extremely uncomfortable during the bimanual examination, particularly with movement of the cervix and uterus **(cervical motion tenderness). Adnexae are tender** to palpation bilaterally, with no palpable mass. **Stool guaiac** is negative.

Labs   Urine **hCG** and **urinalysis** are negative. CBC shows **elevated WBC.** Liver function tests are normal (to rule out **Fitz–Hugh–Curtis syndrome**).

Imaging   Not applicable. (**Ultrasound** is indicated if there is adnexal mass on bimanual examination, severe illness, or inadequate response to appropriate medical therapy.)

Micro Pathology   Microscopic examination of the vaginal discharge shows **gram-negative kidney-shaped diplococci** within the abundant PMNs. A **nucleic acid amplification test** (NAAT) for *Chlamydia* and gonorrhea returns positive for gonorrhea. A cervical culture subsequently confirms *Neisseria gonorrhoeae.*

case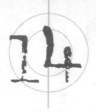

Pelvic Inflammatory Disease

Pathogenesis

Pelvic inflammatory disease (PID), or **acute salpingitis,** is the most common serious complication of sexually transmitted diseases. *Chlamydia trichomatis* and *N. gonorrhoeae* cause a large percentage of PID cases. *C. trichomatis* is especially prevalent in the adolescent and young adult population. However, PID is ultimately a **polymicrobial ascending** infection, such that multiple other organisms, including streptococci, staphylococci, *E. coli, Haemophilus, Klebsiella, Proteus mirabilis, Bacteroides, Peptococcus, Peptostreptococcus, Clostridium,* and *Actinomyces* may also be identified. Risk factors include young age, young age at first intercourse, non-barrier contraception, multiple/new/infected partners, and previous PID.

Epidemiology

Incidence is highest among young females with **multiple sexual partners; unprotected sex** greatly increases the risk of developing PID.

Management

Broad-spectrum antibiotic coverage is necessary at the start of treatment, given the polymicrobial nature of PID, while cultures and sensitivities are pending. Treatment is continued for 10 to 14 days. Various possible antibiotic combinations have been recommended by the CDC, and are summarized in Table 14-1.

Complications

Progression to tubo-ovarian abscess, ectopic pregnancy (6 to 10 times higher risk), infertility, chronic pelvic pain (4 times greater risk), Fitz–Hugh–Curtis syndrome; rarely, sepsis and/or death.

■ **TABLE 14-1 ANTIBIOTIC CHOICES FOR PID**

Oral	Parenteral
Recommended Regimen A	**Recommended Regimen A**
Levofloxacin 500 mg PO daily for 14 days[a]	Cefotetan 2 g IV every 12 hours
OR	**OR**
Ofloxacin 400 mg PO BID for 14 days[a]	Cefoxitin 2 g IV every 6 hours
WITH OR WITHOUT	*PLUS*
Metronidazole 500 mg PO BID for 14 days	Doxycycline 100 mg orally or IV every 12 hours

[a]Based on CDC guidelines 2006, available at http://www.cdc.gov/std/treatment/ 2006/rr5511.pdf.

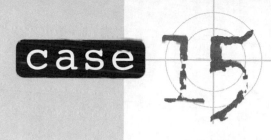

case 15

ID/CC A **20-year-old** woman complains **of inability to conceive, excessive menstrual flow, and bilateral lower abdominal pain.**

HPI She was treated for **pulmonary tuberculosis** a few years ago and has been unable to conceive for the past 2 years. Semen analysis of her husband is normal. She denies cough.

PE VS: normal. PE: **small, fixed adnexal masses** that are **matted and fixed to uterus** ("FROZEN PELVIS"); uterine tenderness; thickening of broad ligament.

Labs CBC: anemia. **Elevated ESR.**

Imaging XR, chest: **cystic cavities and fibrosis** in upper lobes (old, healed pulmonary tuberculosis). Hysterosalpingography (HSG) is contraindicated in a proven case of tuberculosis.

Micro Pathology Culture of endometrial curettage reveals *Mycobacterium tuberculosis*; histologic examination of curettage shows presence of characteristic **granulomas; Mantoux test strongly positive;** ELISA for TB positive.

case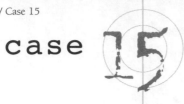

Pelvic Tuberculosis

Pathogenesis

HIV-positive patients are at high risk of developing extrapulmonary TB; therefore, all patients with TB should have counseling about HIV testing. Pelvic tuberculosis usually occurs via hematogenous spread of pulmonary TB. The **fallopian tube** is the most frequently involved part of the genital tract, but can then spread to involve the peritoneum, endometrium, ovaries, cervix, and vagina.

Management

Four-drug therapy with INH, pyrazinamide, ethambutol, and rifampin for 2 months; continue INH and rifampin for another 6 months. **Indications for surgery** include disease progression or persistence despite antibiotic therapy, or formation of tubo-ovarian abscess. Ninety percent **of cases are cured** with intensive therapy, but **only 10% regain fertility.**

Complications

Complications include INH-induced **pyridoxine deficiency** (administer pyridoxine) and **hepatotoxicity** resulting from rifampin and INH (obtain baseline LFTs). **Adhesions** within the uterine cavity form synechiae (ASHERMAN SYNDROME).

Breakout Point

- TB may spread to all sites of the body.
- All active TB cases should be reported to the local health department.

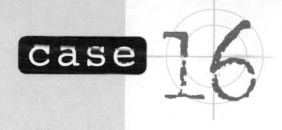

ID/CC	A **26-year-old obese** G0 woman complains of **infertility** for the last 3 years.
HPI	She also complains of intermittent lower abdominal pain and heaviness, as well as lack of menstruation for the past 6 months (**secondary amenorrhea**). Prior to cessation of her menses, she had irregular periods (**metrorrhagia**), occasionally heavy (**menorrhagia**). She also notes excessive facial and body hair (**hirsutism**), as well as acne. She reports family history of irregular periods and infertility, and strong family history of type 2 diabetes mellitus.
PE	VS: normal. PE: **obese**. Increased hair on back and lower abdomen, with stubble on face and arms. **Acne.** Normal breast development; external genitalia normal. Pelvic examination within normal limits. **Acanthosis nigricans** on the axilla and neck.
Labs	**Elevated LH**, low FSH; **increased LH-to-FSH ratio (>3:1)**. Normal prolactin, normal TSH. **Increased free testosterone, DHEA, and androstenedione.** Increased ratio of estrone to estradiol. Glucose testing shows slightly high insulin resistance. Normal estrogen, low progesterone. A progestin challenge test (progesterone given for 5 days) results in a vaginal bleed after the progestin is stopped.
Imaging	US: **multiple small ovarian cysts** bilaterally.

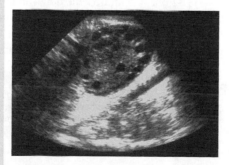

Figure 16-1. US. Note the "string of pearls" small subcortical follicles.

31

case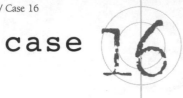

Polycystic Ovarian Disease

Pathogenesis

Polycystic ovary disease (PCOD), also known as **Stein–Leventhal syndrome**, is characterized by irregular periods due to **anovulatory cycles, excess ovarian androgen** production (causing hirsutism and acne), and **multiple ovarian cysts.** Only two of the three characteristics are needed for diagnosis because not all women with PCOD have ultrasound findings of ovarian cysts. Its cause is unclear, but PCOD appears to be familial and strongly associated with insulin resistance. **Obesity** is common, as androstenedione undergoes aromatization to estrone in fat tissue. Estrone stimulates LH and suppresses FSH secretion, which further leads to the vicious cycle of LH causing increased androgen production. Because of anovulatory cycles and lack of progesterone exposure, patients will have unopposed estrogen, causing endometrial hyperplasia and leading to heavy irregular periods.

Epidemiology

PCOD is the **most common cause of hirsutism** and is usually seen in females in their **late teens and young adulthood.**

Management

Weight loss results in symptomatic improvement in many patients, as well as return of menses and ovulation. **Oral contraceptives** increase steroid hormone–binding globulin and suppress the increased LH production, with a consequent decrease in free testosterone and androstenedione, and the return of a regular menstruation. **Metformin** may increase ovulation as well as decrease insulin resistance. **Induction of ovulation** by clomiphene may be attempted for women desiring fertility.

Breakout Point

- PCOD is characterized by irregular periods, increased androgen production, and multiple ovarian cysts.
- Many women with PCOD have infertility.
- PCOD is strongly associated with insulin resistance.

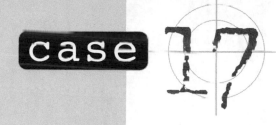

ID/CC   A 33-year-old G3P2011 presents for gynecologic evaluation given her 6-month history of **vaginal spotting after intercourse.**

HPI   She denies any dyspareunia. She also reports occasional **intermenstrual bleeding**. She has had annual Pap smears, which have all been normal.

PE   VS: stable. PE: speculum examination reveals a **2-cm mass protruding from the cervix on a thin stalk.** Contact bleeding is noted from this region when Pap smear is performed. No other cervical lesions are noted. No discharge. The mass is grasped with a Kelly clamp, twisted, and easily removed with excellent hemostasis. Bimanual examination is normal.

Labs   U/A was negative. **Urine hCG is negative.** Gonorrhea and *Chlamydia* cultures are negative.

Gross Pathology   Biopsy of the cervical mass is sent.

Micro Pathology   Pap smear is normal.

case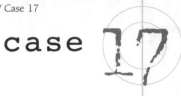

Postcoital Bleeding (Benign Endocervical Polyp)

Pathogenesis Arises within the **endocervical canal** and consists of loose fibromyxomatous stroma containing mucus-secreting endocervical glands often accompanied by inflammation and squamous metaplasia.

Management Based on clinical judgment office removal of polyp if size and stalk are small enough. Alternatively, if lesion or stalk are too large, this may be performed in the OR.

Complications Hemorrhage requiring control with pressure, Monsel solution, or silver nitrate. Infection requiring treatment with antibiotics.

Breakout Point

- Occur in 2% to 5% of women.
- Size varies from small and pedunculated to upwards of 5 cm and sessile.
- Classic symptom is irregular vaginal spotting or bleeding.
- Progression to malignancy is rare.

■ TABLE 17-1 NON–PREGNANCY-RELATED CAUSES OF VAGINAL BLEEDING

Diagnosis	History and Physical Findings	Diagnostic/Confirmatory Tests
Nephrolithiasis	Varied, abd pain, hematuria	Renal ultrasound, cath UA
Cystitis	Varied, abd pain, hematuria	Cath UA
Lower GI tract bleeding	Varied BRBPR, hemorrhoids	Hemoccult testing, PE
Cervical cancer	Vaginal discharge, cervical lesion	Cervical biopsy (not recommended in ED or during pregnancy)
Cervicitis or bacterial vaginosis	Varied, abnormal discharge, pain, spotting	Wet prep, cervical cultures
Cervical ectropion	Postcoital bleeding, friable columnar epithelium seen on endocervical canal	PE
Cervical polyps	Pinkish buds protruding from cervical os	PE
Vaginal wall trauma	Varied	PE

BRBPR, bright red blood per rectum.

case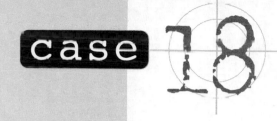

ID/CC	A **24-year-old** G1P1 complains of **mood lability** prior to the onset of her periods.
HPI	Patient's symptoms **correlate well with her menses,** beginning 5 days prior to and **remitting** with the start of her menses. When affected, she feels "**out of control**" and **overwhelmed, irritable**, and **cries** without apparent cause. She reports **symptoms of depression,** including poor sleep, increased appetite, decreased interest in activities (anhedonia), poor concentration, and decreased energy such that she often **misses work** around her menses. She also has **breast tenderness, headache,** and **abdominal bloating** during these episodes. Her menses come in regular intervals of 28 days. She has a previous history of postpartum depression, and smokes one-half pack per day.
PE	VS: normal. A thorough PE is normal.
Labs	CBC, serum chemistries, and TSH are normal.
Imaging	None (if GI symptoms predominate, a KUB or ultra-sound may be appropriate).

■ **TABLE 18-1 KEY ELEMENTS OF A PROSPECTIVE SYMPTOM RECORD TO BE USED FOR THE DIAGNOSIS OF PREMENSTRUAL SYNDROME**

1. Daily listing of symptoms
2. Ratings of symptom severity throughout the month
3. Timing of symptoms in relation to menstruation
4. Rating of baseline symptom severity during the follicular phase

case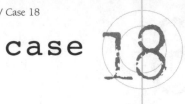

Premenstrual Dysphoric Disorder

Pathogenesis
Premenstrual dysphoric disorder (PMD) is thought to occur when *normal* fluctuations in estrogen and progesterone cause an *abnormal* change in CNS neurotransmitter levels or neurotransmitter receptor activity. **Serotonin** in particular seems to have a strong relationship to PMD. Some opioid pathways, GABA, and the autonomic nervous system may also be affected by hormonal levels and be responsible for some of the systemic manifestations, such as GI symptoms. No significant personality or stress factors have been found to cause PMD.

Epidemiology
Premenstrual dysphoric disorder is seen in 2% to 6% of the population. Genetic predisposition (family history) may play a role. Higher frequency seen in patients with **preexisting depression** and those who suffered from **postpartum depression.**

Management
PMD is a diagnosis of exclusion, so other causes of symptoms must be ruled out. The patient should **chart her symptoms prospectively** for at least two cycles before the diagnosis of PMD is given formally. **Exercise,** reducing sodium intake (to reduce edema), NSAIDs, and pyridoxine and magnesium supplements may improve symptoms; avoidance of caffeine and cigarettes is also recommended. **SSRIs** (fluoxetine, paroxetine, citalopram, sertraline) and/or counseling may be used for depressive symptoms. "Medical oophorectomy" with **GnRH agonists** is effective for physical symptoms, but is not effective for depressive symptoms. This also effectively causes menopause, and patients can experience hot flashes, night sweats, irritability, and bone density loss. GnRH agonist treatment is not recommended for more than 3 to 6 months at a time because of the hypoestrogenic effects. If hormone add-back therapy is given, GnRH agonist treatment is safe for up to 12 months.

Breakout Point

- Key to diagnosis is the presence of a "disease-free period" during the follicular phase of the menstrual cycle.
- The diagnosis of PMD requires that the symptoms interfere with life (work, school, social activities, or relationships with others).
- 30% to 76% of women with PMD have a history of depression.

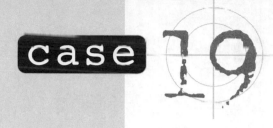

ID/CC A 20-year-old woman presents for an evaluation of **amenorrhea.**

HPI She has **never menstruated.** She complains of **swelling in the inguinal and labial region.**

PF **Tall** with **eunuchoid features; large breasts,** but with sparse glandular tissue; nipples and areolae pale; **no axillary or pubic hair; bilateral inguinal hernias (containing ectopic testes);** slightly underdeveloped labia minora; vagina ends as **blind pouch.**

Labs Karyotype: **46,XY.** Serum **testosterone levels normal for male.**

Imaging US: **absent uterus and rudimentary fallopian tubes;** no ovaries.

Gross Pathology Bilateral small testes removed during bilateral inguinal herniorrhaphy.

Micro Pathology Biopsy of removed testes reveals **no evidence of spermatogenesis.** No evidence of malignancy.

case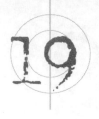

Primary Amenorrhea—Androgen Insensitivity

Pathogenesis

Androgen insensitivity (previously called testicular feminization) is inherited as an **X-linked recessive trait** resulting in the **absence of androgen receptors**; individuals have a 46,XY genotype and a female phenotype. Because müllerian inhibiting factor is secreted, these individuals have an absence of müllerian-derived structures.

Epidemiology

The incidence of primary amenorrhea is <3%. Androgen insensitivity is the third most common cause (accounting for approximately 10% of all cases). This follows gonadal dysgenesis (#1) and congenital absence of the uterus and vagina (#2).

Management

Patients are usually regarded socially as **female**; **gonadectomy** is performed because of the increased risk (50%) of **testicular neoplasia. Estrogen treatment** is given for maintaining secondary sexual characteristics. Surgical treatment involves **creation of a vagina.**

Complications

Confused gender identity and infertility.

Breakout Point

- Patients with androgen insensitivity are referred to as male hermaphrodites.
- Genotypically male, phenotypically female.
- Deficiency or defect of androgen receptor.
- Breast development is normal because high levels of testosterone are aromatized to estradiol.
- Pubic and axillary hair are sparse (dependent on androgen activity)
- Gonadectomy is performed because of increased risk of testicular neoplasia.

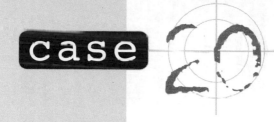

case 20

ID/CC	A 17-year-old girl is brought by her mother to a gynecologist because her **periods have not yet begun** (PRIMARY AMENORRHEA).
HPI	She underwent surgical repair for **coarctation of the aorta** a few years ago.
PE	VS: normal. PE: **short in stature, low-set ears**; absence of breasts, pubic and axillary hair; external genitalia not well developed; **short, webbed neck; shield chest** with widely spaced nipples; increased **carrying angle at elbow** (CUBITUS VALGUS).
Labs	**Low estradiol; high pituitary gonadotropins** (hypergonadotropic hypergonadism). Karyotype: **45,XO.**
Imaging	Pelvic ultrasound: **"streak" ovaries.**

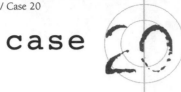

case

Primary Amenorrhea (Turner Syndrome)

Pathogenesis

Most patients with Turner syndrome have a **45,XO karyotype;** others have an alteration in the structure of one of the X chromosomes or exhibit a **mosaic pattern** for two or more cell lines (usually 45,X and either 46,XY or 46,XX). A mosaic pattern will result in various degrees of **gonadal dysgenesis, secondary amenorrhea, and premature menopause;** if a Y chromosome is present in the genotype, the risk of **gonadoblastomas** makes gonadectomy advisable. Turner syndrome is associated with coarctation of the aorta.

Epidemiology

Incidence is 1 in 2,500 live female births. Gonadal dysgenesis (Turner syndrome and its mosaic variants) is the leading cause of primary amenorrhea, accounting for approximately 30% to 40% of all cases.

Management

To increase potential height, short stature can be treated with **oxandrolone** (an anabolic steroid) **and/or growth hormone.** Subsequently, **estrogen replacement therapy** is usually initiated around age 12 to 13 to stimulate development of secondary sexual characteristics. Cyclical use of estrogen and progesterone will initiate regular menstrual bleeding, although infertility persists.

Complications

Gonadal neoplasia and infertility.

Breakout Point

- Due to ovarian failure, LH and FSH are elevated because of the lack of estrogen's negative feedback on the HPA (hypothalamus-pituitary-adrenal) axis.
- Most Turner syndrome patients lack secondary sexual characteristics and have primary amenorrhea.

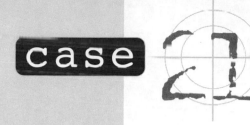

ID/CC A 20-year-old G0 college student is brought to the ER after being found by campus security lying in the bushes outside her dorm.

HPI The patient is dazed and does not speak. Her roommate states she called campus security this morning when the patient did not return from a party they attended at a fraternity the night before. The patient, once coherent, only remembers drinking a fruity cocktail handed to her by one of her hosts; she does not recall much of the events that followed.

PE VS: normal. PE: her clothes are disheveled and her underwear is missing. Her throat, breasts, and arms show abrasions and contusions, and her inner thighs reveal more contusions and streaks of dried blood and semen. Her vulva is swollen and excoriated, and her hymenal ring has a posterior laceration.

Labs CBC: normal. RPR/HIV: negative. UA: mild hematuria. Samples from throat, anus, and vagina sent for Gram stain and gonococcal and *Chlamydia* culture; pregnancy test negative. γ-Hydroxybutyrate (GHB) test is positive.

Imaging CXR: normal. Head CT: normal.

Micro Pathology Gonorrhea, *Chlamydia*, and wet prep tests negative.

■ **TABLE 21-1 BASIC SEXUAL ASSAULT TREATMENT PROTOCOL**

1. Obtain an accurate and thorough medical and gynecologic history, including details of the assault.
2. Assess, document, and treat physical injuries.
3. Obtain appropriate cultures and forensic sampling; treat any existing infection and provide STD prophylaxis.
4. Offer HIV and pregnancy prophylaxis.
5. Provide counseling to the patient and her family.
6. Arrange for appropriate follow-up care.
7. Report to legal authorities in accordance with state law.

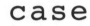 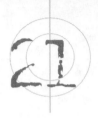

Rape/Sexual Assault

Pathogenesis

Sexual assault requires three key elements: **threat or the use of force, evidence of sexual contact with or without penetration, and lack of effective consents.** Rape is forced sexual acts which are either physical or psychological.

Epidemiology

Only an estimated 10% to 15% of all rapes will be reported to police. 50% of rapists are known to the victim (an acquaintance or spouse). One in three women will be sexually assaulted sometime in her life. One in four will experience rape or attempted rape during her college years. 7–10% of rape victims are male.

Management

Victims of sexual violence have medical, forensic, and psychosocial care needs. A detailed history should be taken, including relevant obstetric and gynecologic data such as **last date of coitus** (to aid in semen analysis) and **last menstrual period.** A careful PE should be completed, including photographs of injuries taken with the patient's consent. **A Wood lamp or other UV lighting** will allow semen or other debris to be seen. Particulate matter should be collected as evidence (the victim's clothing, fngernail scrapings and clippings, scalp and pubic hair combings and cuttings). Obtain swabs and smears from the mouth, anus, vagina. **Testing and labs** include cultures for gonococcus and *Chlamydia*; wet prep to examine for bacterial vaginosis, trichomonas, and motile sperm; baseline pregnancy, hepatitis B, syphilis and HIV (voluntary) tests. Prophylactic treatments to offer include tetanus, hepatitis B, and HIV-exposure prophylaxis; ceftriaxone and doxycycline or azithromycin for gonorrhea and *Chlamydia*; metronidazole for trichomoniasis; and postcoital emergency contraception.

Complications

The rape-trauma syndrome consists of immediate and chronic phases. In the immediate phase, a victim may experience severe mood swings and feelings of anger, fear, guilt, disbelief, pain, and denial. In the second phase, a victim may experience nightmares and relationship difficulties, which may be indicative of PTSD. Other complications include STD infection, HIV, and pregnancy.

Breakout Point

- Rape is defined as any sexual act performed by one person on another without consent.
- The majority of rape and sexual assaults are not reported, and are often committed by someone the victim knows.

case

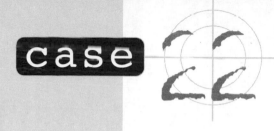

ID/CC   A 35-year-old G1P1001 woman complains of **galactorrhea, visual feld deficits, and inability to conceive.**

HPI   The patient has been **amenorrheic** for the past 6 months and also feels that her **field of vision** is **constricted**; she denies use of any medications or drugs. She has a healthy 7-year-old son (SECONDARY INFERTILITY), has not been using any contraceptives for 2 years, and wishes to conceive.

PE   Visual-field charting reveals **bitemporal hemianopsia**; pelvic examination is unremarkable; **breasts express milk** readily with pressure.

Labs   Pregnancy test negative; **TSH normal; elevated prolactin** (850 ng/mL); breast biopsy normal.

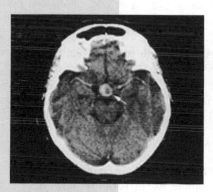

Figure 22-1. Head CT, coronal: Enhancing pituitary adenoma (>10 mm) compressing the optic chiasm.

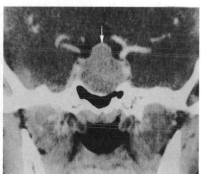

Figure 22-2. Pituitary macrodenoma.

case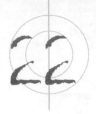

Secondary Amenorrhea (Prolactinoma)

Pathogenesis

Hyperprolactinemia is defned as a prolactin level of >20 ng/mL and is considered signifcant when accompanied by oligomenorrhea. Hyperprolactinemia interferes with the menstrual cycle by suppressing the pulsatility of LH release from the pituitary; common causes include **prolactinoma, primary hypothyroidism, drugs** such as metoclopramide and phenothiazines, and **chronic renal failure.** It may also be **idiopathic.**

Epidemiology

Pituitary microadenomas (size <10 mm) are quite common and present in 10% to 30% of patients at autopsy. Macroadenomas (size >10 mm) are more likely to be diagnosed during life as they tend to be more clinically relevant.

Management

Bromocriptine (dopamine agonist) to attempt to decrease size of tumor and mass effect, followed by **surgical** resection if symptoms persist despite medical management or if the tumor does not decrease in size; **fertility is usually restored** after treatment. For tumors <10 mm (microadenomas), bromocriptine and surveillance imaging with periodic head MRIs. If menses do not resume, ovulation induction may be achieved with clomiphene citrate.

Complications

Infertility and panhypopituitarism.

Breakout Point

- The anterior pituitary secretes prolactin, growth hormone, ACTH, TSH, FSH, and LH.
- The posterior pituitary secretes vasopressin (antidiuretic hormone) and oxytocin.
- Secondary amenorrhea occurs because elevated prolactin inhibits pulsatile GnRH, subsequently decreasing FSH and LH secretion.

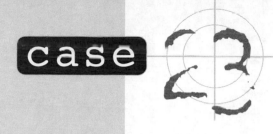

case 23

ID/CC	A 38-year-old female smoker presents with **right leg swelling** and tenderness.
HPI	No recent leg trauma, no shortness of breath. She has been **taking oral contraceptives** for approximately 4 years.
PE	VS normal. Lungs are clear to auscultation. The right leg is larger and warmer than the left. Palpable cord in right leg, with positive Homan sign.
Labs	CBC: increased hematocrit and hemoglobin (chronic smoker). D-dimer is elevated.
Imaging	Doppler US shows a right-sided deep venous thrombus. CT angiogram shows no pulmonary embolus.

case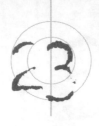

Side Effects of Oral Contraception

Pathogenesis

Cerebrovascular accidents (CVAs), deep venous thrombosis (DVT), and **pulmonary embolism** are more common in OCP users than in nonusers. This may be due to intimal and medial vascular injury, increased platelet aggregation, and a decrease in antithrombin III activity and plasminogen activator caused by the estrogen component of the pill. The effect is dose dependent; with reduction in the estrogen content of the pill, the incidence of thromboembolic disorders falls. The combination of **oral contraception in a >35-year-old smoker** represents the "classic" high-risk patient for DVT development. Other risk factors are described by the Virchow triangle: hypercoagulable state, stasis, and endothelial injury.

Management

Discontinue OCPs. Treat with initial unfractionated **heparin** or low–molecular-weight heparin, then transition to **warfarin**. Warfarin is continued for 6 months in uncomplicated patients. When applicable, counsel the patient to stop smoking.

Breakout Point

> OCPs are contraindicated in:
> - Age >35 years and smoke >15 cigarettes per day.
> - History of thromboembolic disease.
> - Concurrent breast, liver, endometrial cancer
> - Completed term pregnancy within 10–14 days

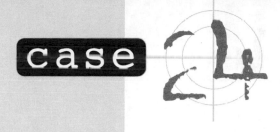

case 24

ID/CC A 27-year-old homeless woman presents to a community health clinic with a **diffuse rash.**

HPI The rash began several months ago as faint, flat **(macular)** lesions on her trunk and arms, and has **evolved** into a **diffuse, raised, occasionally pustular,** painless rash that now involves her **palms and soles.** She reports having a moist, raised lesion around her anus **(condyloma lata)** a few weeks ago that she assumed was a wart, but has since resolved. She denies **neurologic deficits,** including visual or auditory changes. She comes in today because of her ongoing **fever, headache, anorexia, and myalgias.**

PE VS: normal. She has a **polymorphic, diffuse, "coppery" papular rash** on her trunk, arms, **palms, and soles.** She also has lesions on her face along the hairline **(corona veneris).** Her scalp has multiple 2-cm to 4-cm areas of alopecia that have a **"moth-eaten"** appearance. She has **generalized nontender lymphadenopathy** involving her cervical, axillary, and inguinal lymph nodes. Rest of examination is normal.

Labs RPR (a nontreponemal test) is positive to a titer of 1:32 (this is a rapid, nonspecific screening test). **FTA-ABS/MHA-TP** (treponemal test) is also positive.

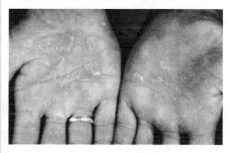

Figure 24-1. Papulosquamous lesions on the palms.

case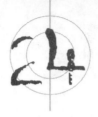

Syphilis

Pathogenesis

Syphilis is caused by a systemic infection by *Treponema pallidum*, a spirochete. The screening test for syphilis is the **rapid plasma reagin (RPR)** test, also known as the **Venereal Disease Research Laboratory (VDRL)** test. RPR is a rapid test that checks for antibodies produced in reaction to syphilis infection. The diagnostic treponemal tests are the **microhemagglutination assay for *T. pallidum*** (MHA-TP) and the **fluorescent treponemal antibody absorption (FTA-ABS)** test; however, the treponemal titers do not correlate with disease severity or treatment response. Treatment response instead should be tracked with RPR/VDRL. Syphilis is most often transmitted via direct contact with infectious lesion (chancre, mucous patch, condyloma latum). In utero or perinatal transmission to neonates can also occur. **Primary syphilis** is characterized by a painless ulcer (**chancre**) that develops 10 to 60 days after infection and heals spontaneously in 3 to 9 weeks. **Secondary syphilis** develops 4 to 8 weeks after the appearance of the chancre. **Early latent** (first year of infection) and **late latent** (>1 year of infection) are asymptomatic periods of time. Approximately one third of patients then progress to **tertiary syphilis** (1 to 20 years after initial infection), characterized by **gummas** (destructive granulomas), **tabes dorsalis** (posterior column degeneration), **Argyll–Robertson pupil** (accommodates but does not react to light), and aortitis.

Management

Penicillin is the primary treatment. Sexual partners of patients should be offered testing.

Complications

Condylomata lata (highly infective mucous lesions, which resolve spontaneously in 2 to 6 weeks), meningitis, hepatitis, and nephritis may also be seen in secondary syphilis. Presence of genital lesions increases the risk of acquiring HIV infection.

Breakout Point

- Primary syphilis, with painless chancres on genitalia, mouth, or anus, often goes unnoticed.
- Coinfection with HIV makes severe complications more likely, and possibly harder to treat.
- **Treponemal** tests will stay positive even after adequate treatment. VDRL is a **reaginic** test like RPR, and titers for both should decrease with treatment.

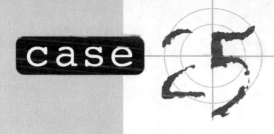

ID/CC An **11-year old girl** comes to the clinic for her annual checkup. She wonders when she will go through **puberty.**

HPI She is otherwise **healthy** without any **nutritional deficiencies.** She is not sexually active. Note: by the age of about 10, the girl or teenager should be seen alone, as this allows her to ask questions without parental interference.

PE The developmental milestones of a girl through pre-puberty or puberty include assessment of breast and pubic hair development, height spurt, and onset of menarche. If a teenage girl is not sexually active and has no anatomic abnormalities or gynecologic complaints, then a pelvic examination is usually not necessary until she is 18.

Labs Labs are not necessary when a girl is developing normally.

■ **TABLE 25-1 FEMALE TANNER STAGES**

Tanner Stage	Development	Female Breast	Female Pubic Hair
1	Prepubertal	Papillae elevated	Vellus hair only
2	Onset age 8–13	Breast buds and papillae elevated	Sparse, long, dark hair on labia only
3	Menarche occurs at about age 12	Breasts and areola enlargement	Extension of more curly and thicker hair to mons pubis
4	Peak of growth	Nipple and areola form secondary mound	Adult hair pattern but less abundant with no extension to medial thigh
5		Areola merges with breast contour, projected nipple only, mature	Adult hair pattern with spread to medial thigh

case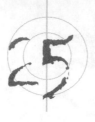

Tanner Stages

Pathogenesis

Tanner stages define the **sequence of secondary sexual characteristic development,** and are useful as a guide. The progression of prepuberty and puberty is divided into several stages. **Adrenarche** (i.e., adrenal gland) occurs between ages 6 and 10, and is characterized by increasing secretions of androgens by the adrenal cortex. **Gonadarche** (i.e., gonad, or ovaries) is characterized by hypothalamic pulsatile GnRH secretion, which stimulates the secretion of LH and FSH by the anterior pituitary, resulting in growth of the ovaries and production of estradiol. **Thelarche,** development of breast buds around age 11, and **pubarche,** development of pubic hair around age 12, represent the first stages in which phenotypic signs of puberty can be seen. Female adolescents can attain their growth spurts between the ages of 12 and 13, up to 2 years ahead of their male counterparts. **Menarche** refers to the onset of menstruation, which occurs around age 12 to 13.

Management

Not relevant.

Complications

Not relevant.

Breakout Point

- Menstruation is usually irregular after onset of menarche for 6 months to up to 2 years, representing anovulatory cycles.
- Primary amenorrhea is defined as absence of menses at age 16 in the presence of normal development of secondary sexual characteristics.
- A variation of one Tanner stage difference, sometimes two, can be normal and is not an indicator of delayed maturation.

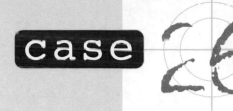
ID/CC A **30-year-old** woman complains a feeling of **lower abdominal pressure** of 4 months' duration.

HPI She is nulliparous and has never used any contraception. Her last menstrual period was 1 week ago. No weight loss or anorexia.

PE VS: normal. PE: well hydrated, thin, and in no acute distress; soft, **rounded, nontender right lower quadrant mass**; bimanual palpation confirms **enlarged right adnexa** with freely **mobile** 7-cm mass located anterior to broad ligament; cervix appears normal.

Labs CBC/Lytes: normal. TFTs, PT/PTT, and INR: normal. UA: normal. Pregnancy test negative. AFP and LDH are normal.

Imaging Ultrasound shows a hyperechoic nodule (with distal acoustic shadowing) within a large multicystic right ovarian mass. Pelvic CT show a multicystic mass containing teeth.

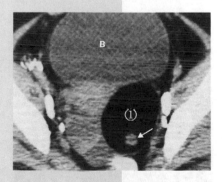

Figure 26-1. CT, pelvis: an oval-shaped mass (*1*) with the same density as fat is seen posterior to the bladder (*B*) and has an area of hyperdensity (*arrow*) within.

case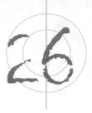

Teratoma

Pathogenesis

Mature teratomas are **germ cell tumors** derived from ectodermal differentiation of totipotential cells and are **usually benign**. They may contain hair, cartilage, thyroid, nervous tissue, teeth, and skin (**three germ cell layers:** ectoderm, mesoderm, and endoderm) and may attain a size of up to 20 cm. When the ectodermal component is prominent, it is termed a dermoid cyst; the most common ovarian tumor in children. Immature teratomas are malignant.

Management

Surgical removal of teratoma allows definitive diagnosis, preservation of part of the ovary, and prevents possible complications of torsion and rupture. Explore the contralateral ovary in view of the risk of bilaterality. Recurrence is rare.

Breakout Point

- Most common in 2nd and 3rd decades of life.
- Symptoms may also include torsion (usually if teratoma is large) and rupture (which may cause hemorrhage and shock).
- Malignant transformation in 1% of mature teratomas.

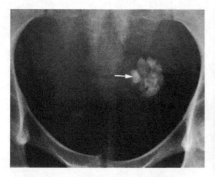

Figure 26-2. XR, pelvis: another case demonstrates teeth (*arrow*) within the cyst.

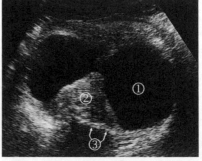

Figure 26-3. US, pelvis: another case shows a mixed cystic (*1*) and solid (*2*) mass with areas of calcification (*3*) due to teeth inside the cyst.

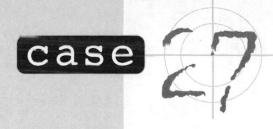

case 27

ID/CC A 17-year-old girl presents to the emergency room with **abrupt-onset high fever, vomiting, diarrhea, and headache** for the past day.

HPI She has since developed a rash, an achy feeling in her muscles (**myalgias**), and dizziness with standing (**orthostasis**). She is on her **third day of menstruation** through which she has used **tampons** exclusively; last tampon was placed nearly 24 hours before.

PE VS: **tachycardia** (HR 110), **fever** (39.2°C), and **hypotension** (systolic pressure <90). PE: toxic-appearing; drowsy but following commands. **Diffuse macular erythroderma** ("sunburn" appearance) seen over her trunk, arms, and hands. **Pharyngeal and conjunctival, mucosa congestion** is noted. Abdomen with hyperactive bowel sounds, no hepatosplenomegaly, no rebound/guarding, and guaiac negative. Pelvic examination significant for a **tampon** only slightly bloody; no active bleeding from the cervical os. Vaginal mucosa is hyperemic and congested. No neck rigidity or Kernig sign; no localizing neurologic deficit found.

Labs CBC: **leukocytosis, anemia,** and **thrombocytopenia** (<100,000). UA: mild pyuria. Elevated BUN and creatinine, **CPK, bilirubin, AST,** and **ALT. Low albumin. Blood culture negative for growth;** vaginal cultures yield *Staphylococcus aureus*. LP: CSF normal.

case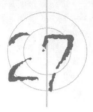

Staphylococcal Toxic Shock Syndrome

Pathogenesis

Staphylococcal TSS is caused by an *S. aureus* infection, and symptoms are mediated through the **exotoxin TSST-1**, a **superantigen** that stimulates a massive T-cell proliferation and cytokine release (including **interleukin-1 and -2, tumor necrosis factor,** and **interferon-gamma**). Because the disease is caused by toxins, blood cultures are usually negative for growth. Some endotoxins have also been associated with TSS. Lack of antibodies to TSST-1 increases susceptibility to TSS. **Super-absorbent tampons** obstruct menstrual outflow, causing retrograde flow and peritoneal seeding with bacteria.

Epidemiology

Staphylococcal TSS can occur at any age, though most cases occur in young, menstruating women. Nonmenstrual causes include postsurgical wound infections, infections of the sinuses or soft tissue, burns, or superinfections of the respiratory tract following the flu.

Management

Patients with TSS require immediate treatment of hypotension and shock with **aggressive fluid resuscitation and vasopressors,** if needed. The offending foreign body and wound should be removed (e.g., tampon removal, drainage of any staphylococcal abscesses). The role of antibiotics is unclear, but β-**lactamase–resistant penicillin** or a **cephalosporin** is ideal. **Clindamycin** reduces protein (i.e., TSST-1 and endotoxin) synthesis in vitro and is often administered concomitantly.

Complications

Acute complications include acute respiratory distress syndrome, cardiac dysrhythmia, DIC with thrombocytopenia, and shock with end-organ failure. There is a 2% to 3% mortality rate.

Breakout Point

- The key is **rapid onset** of **severe illness** in an **otherwise healthy** individual.
- May occur with any foreign material (e.g., diaphragm, contraceptive sponges) left in the vagina for too long, leading to *S. aureus* colonization.

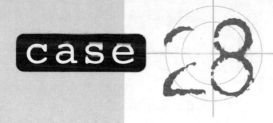
case 28

ID/CC A 30-year-old G4P4 presents to the gynecologist's office to discuss surgical sterilization.

HPI The patient is happily married, with children ranging from 12 months to 6 years of age. She and her husband want no more children. Patient is otherwise healthy.

PE VS: normal. Thorough PE reveals no abnormal finding.

case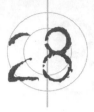

Tubal Ligation

Pathogenesis

By **occluding the fallopian tubes,** surgical sterilization **prevents fertilization of the ovum by sperm.** Occlusion may be accomplished by banding, clipping, electrocautery, or tubal ligation (most commonly, the Pomeroy method), and requires general anesthesia. Failure rate (i.e., pregnancy despite surgical sterilization) is <1%.

Management

The physician should counsel the patient on the permanent nature of tubal ligation, risks of the operation and general anesthesia, and chance of failure. Side effects of tubal ligation are minimal. After surgical sterilization, about 1% of women will seek reversal. The success of reversal ranges from 40% to 50% (electrocautery and Pomeroy procedure) to 70% to 80% (clips and bands).

Complications

The risk of operative mortality is about 4 in 100,000. Risk of ectopic pregnancy is about 1 in 15,000.

Breakout Point

- Surgical sterilization does not prevent sexually transmitted diseases.

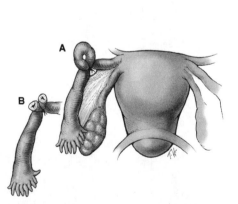

Figure 28-1. Pomeroy technique for tubal sterilization.

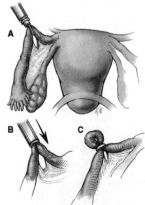

Figure 28-2. Placement of Falope ring for tubal sterilization.

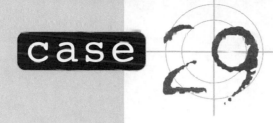

case

ID/CC	A 23-year-old woman complains of **fever** and **intense abdominal pain** for the past few days.
HPI	She had unprotected intercourse with a new partner 5 days ago. She denies any history of sexually transmitted disease. Her last period was 1 week ago.
PE	VS: Temperature 102.5°F. Abdominal examination reveals diffuse tenderness in the lower quadrants, right greater than left, with rebound and guarding. Pelvic examination is significant for cervical motion tenderness and a palpable **adnexal mass**.
Labs	WBC 23 with a left shift. Urine hCG negative. Urinalysis negative. Liver function tests normal.
Imaging	Pelvic ultrasound shows a right **adnexal mass** with **thick, irregular septations** and a **thickened echogenic wall**.
Micro Pathology	Cervical specimen positive for *Chlamydia trachomatis*. Culture of abscess reveals mixed flora, including *Bacteroides*.

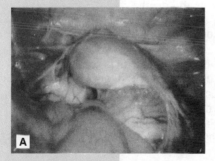
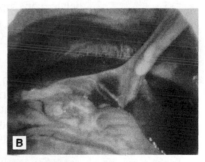

Figure 29-1. (A) Filmy adhesions from resolved PID. Bilateral ovarian cysts are also seen. **(B)** Evidence of Fitz Hugh-Curtis syndrome, with violin-string–like adhesions between the liver and the anterior abdominal wall.

case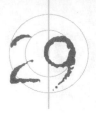

Tubo-ovarian Abscess

Pathogenesis

Persistent pelvic inflammatory disease results in the formation of a tubo-ovarian abscess (TOA), as the host immunity attempts to isolate the infection. It is estimated that 10% to 15% of PID cases progress to form a TOA. Thus, when a patient being treated for PID is not improving symptomatically, further workup is necessary to rule out TOA formation.

Management

Patients need to be hospitalized for management. Standard treatment includes **abscess drainage,** by either transvaginal approach or laparoscopy, with concurrent **broad-spectrum antibiotics,** particularly targeted against anaerobes. Patient course is closely followed with serial examinations and by watching the trending of patient temperature and WBC counts. There are some clinicians who manage TOAs conservatively with antibiotics only, for patients in whom the abscess has not ruptured (i.e., no peritoneal signs), although this is controversial.

Complications

Tubal rupture with hemorrhage, Fitz–Hugh–Curtis syndrome, infertility, ectopic pregnancy, chronic pelvic pain, sepsis, and death.

Breakout Point

- TOA is considered the most severe form of PID.
- Although gonorrhea and *Chlamydia* are often initiating organisms for PID, anaerobic coverage is crucial in antibiotics for treating TOA.
- A patient diagnosed with TOA must be initially managed as an inpatient because of the high risk of tubal rupture and/or sepsis.

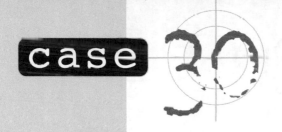

case 30

ID/CC	A 47-year-old G4P4 woman presents with **involuntary leakage of urine** for the past few years.
HPI	She states her symptoms are precipitated by **coughing, sneezing, and exercise,** and she needs to wear a pad daily. She reports no urgency or frequency. She denies dysuria or hematuria. A **bladder voiding diary** confirms two to three episodes of incontinence per day. Obstetric history is notable for four spontaneous vaginal deliveries.
PE	VS: normal. Pelvic examination reveals normal external female genitalia. Mild pelvic relaxation is noted; however, no pelvic organ prolapse is observed. Q-tip test (insertion of cotton-tip applicator inside urethra) confirms **urethral hypermobility** by demonstrating **>30° change with Valsalva maneuver.** Immediate leakage of urine can be observed with vigorous cough with the patient in the standing position. Postvoid residual volume is normal.
Labs	Urinalysis and urine culture negative.

■ TABLE 30-1 BASIC TYPES AND CAUSES OF URINARY INCONTINENCE

Type	Symptoms	Common Causes
Stress	Involuntary loss of urine (usually small amounts) simultaneous with increases in intra-abdominal pressure, such as those caused by coughing, laughing, and changing positions. Severe stress incontinence may be manifested by constant wetting.	Weakness and laxity of pelvic floor musculature resulting in hypermobility of the bladder base and proximal urethra.
		Bladder outlet or urethral sphincter weakness (intrinsic sphincter deficiency) related to prior surgery or trauma.
Urge	Leakage of urine (usually larger, but often variable, volumes) because of inability to delay voiding after sensation of bladder fullness is perceived.	Bladder hyperactivity isolated or associated with one or more of the following.
		Local genitourinary condition, such as cystitis, urethritis, tumors, stones, diverticula, outflow obstruction; impaired bladder contractability. CNS disorders, such as stroke, dementia, parkinsonism, spinal cord injury or disease.
Overflow	Leakage of urine (usually small amounts) resulting from mechanical forces on an overdistended bladder. May present similar to stress and urge incontinence.	Anatomic obstruction by prostate, or large cystocele that kinks the urethra.
		A contractile bladder associated with diabetes mellitus or low spinal cord injury.
Functional[a]	Urinary leakage associated with inability to toilet because of impairment of cognitive or physical functioning, psychological unwillingness, or environmental barriers.	Severe dementia, immobility, physical restraints, inaccessible toilets, unavailability of regular toileting assistance, depression.

[a]Functional incontinence should be a diagnosis of exclusion. Many frail geriatric patients have functional factors that may contribute to incontinence but may also have reversible and specifically treatable conditions underlying the incontinence.

case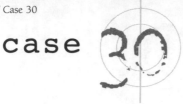

Urinary Incontinence

Pathogenesis

Stress urinary incontinence is defined as the involuntary leakage of urine with increases in intra-abdominal pressure during **physical exertion involving Valsalva maneuvers** (running, bending, coughing, sneezing, or laughing). During these episodes, **intravesical pressure exceeds the maximum urethral closure pressure in the absence of a detrusor contraction.** Risk factors for the development of urinary incontinence include childbirth, obesity, aging, and genitourinary surgery. Urethral support becomes impaired because of weakening of the pelvic fascia and musculature.

Management

Conservative measures should be undertaken prior to consideration of surgical intervention. **Lifestyle changes** include avoiding caffeinated beverages and alcohol, and treating potential aggravating factors such as coughing or constipation. **Behavioral modification techniques and pelvic floor muscle training (Kegel exercises)** are valuable components of therapy for these patients. Pharmacologic therapy is helpful for patients with urge incontinence, but does not play a meaningful role in symptomatic relief for patients with stress urinary incontinence. If these methods fail for a patient who wishes to avoid surgery, **pessaries** are a reasonable option. If patients do not respond to conservative therapy, surgical procedures such as **bladder neck suspension or sling procedures** may be warranted.

Complications

Complications are infrequent and typically mild. Symptoms may cause **significant disruption in daily activities.**

Breakout Point

- Stress urinary incontinence represents the most common type of incontinence in younger women.
- Leakage with stress maneuvers is a very sensitive finding for stress urinary incontinence.

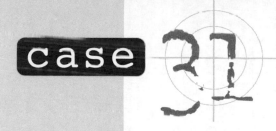
case

ID/CC	A 27-year-old recently married woman complains of **frequent** and painful urination (**dysuria**).
HPI	The patient just returned from her honeymoon. She also reports urinary **urgency**, and is able to void only small volumes. She experiences burning with urination and has some **suprapubic pain**.
PE	VS: normal. Mild suprapubic tenderness. No costovertebral angle or flank tenderness.
Labs	Urinalysis shows positive leukocyte esterase and nitrites.
Micro Pathology	Urine microscopy shows 50 WBC, 5 RBC, and many bacteria per high-powered field. Urine culture grows out 100,000 colonies of pan-sensitive *E. coli*.

▦ TABLE 31-1 ANTIBIOTIC REGIMENS FOR URINARY TRACT INFECTIONS

Clinical Situation	Regimen
Acutely ill and toxic patient	Hospitalization; parenteral antibiotics; ampicillin plus gentamicin if urosepsis suspected; otherwise, ciprofloxacin if Gram stain shows GNR; ampicillin if it shows GPC
Uncomplicated pyelonephritis	Oral TMS (1 double-strength tablet) bid for 2 wk or ciprofloxacin 500 mg bid for 2 wk
Uncomplicated lower UTI	Single-dose TMS (2 double-strength tablets), ciprofloxacin (1 g), or amoxicillin (3 g) if Gram stain shows GNR; amoxicillin if it shows GPC; 3-day course if more symptomatic with TMS (1 double-strength tablet) bid, ciprofloxacin 500 mg bid, amoxicillin 500 mg tid; 7–10-day course if diabetes, recurrent UTI, age >65 yr
Relapse	Same drug as for uncomplicated UTI, but continued for at least 2 wk
Acute urethral syndrome with pyuria	TMS as for uncomplicated UTI or doxycycline 100 mg bid for 10 days if *Chlamydia* infection suspected
Acute urethral syndrome without pyuria	No antibiotics
Recurrent infection	
Sexually active	Prophylaxis with nocturnal single-tablet dose of ampicillin, TMS, or ciprofloxacin
Elderly patient with large postvoid residual	Prophylaxis with nightly dose of TMS (half of a single-strength tablet) or ciprofloxacin (250 mg)
Pregnancy	Ampicillin, amoxicillin, and oral cephalosporins have proved to be safe; nitrofurantoin is safe for the fetus but potentially toxic for the mother; fluoroquinolones should be avoided

GNR, gram-negative rod; GPC, gram-positive cocci; TMS, trimethoprim/sulfamethoxazole; UTI, urinary tract infection.

case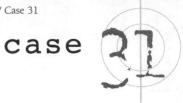

Urinary Tract Infection

Pathogenesis

The urinary tract can be contaminated by **fecal bacteria that ascend via the urethra.** Such infections may remain in the lower tract (urethritis, cystitis) or may ascend further to the upper tract (pyelonephritis). The most common causative organisms of urinary tract infections (UTIs) are **E. coli,** *Proteus, Klebsiella,* enterococci, and *Pseudomonas.* UTIs are more common in women than in men, because of a shorter urethra, and can be seen with the onset of frequent sexual activity, because of both mechanical factors and the use of lubricants/spermicides.

Management

For an **uncomplicated UTI,** antibiotic treatment with TMP-SMZ (Bactrim), a fluoroquinolone, or a broad-spectrum cephalosporin for 3 days is usually sufficient. Asymptomatic bacteriuria in a pregnant woman should also be treated. Diabetics should be treated for a week. **Complicated UTIs** (pregnant women or upper tract infection or patients with underlying structural or neurologic disease) should be treated for 10 to 14 days. If the patient experiences significant pain with voiding, a short course of **phenazopyridine** may be added, although this may mask signs of recurrent infection if used for more than a few days.

Complications

Untreated lower UTI can ascend to upper urinary tract, causing more serious infections such as pyelonephritis. This risk is even higher in pregnant women; therefore, patients must be treated during pregnancy even in the absence of symptoms. Like any infection, UTI can cause preterm contractions during pregnancy.

Breakout Point

- Overall most common cause of UTI is *E. Coli.*
- Most common cause of UTI in female adolescents is Staphylococcus saprophytieus.

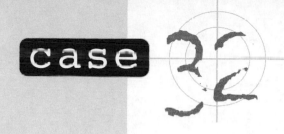

case 32

ID/CC	A 35-year-old woman presents with **blood-stained discharge from the left nipple,** and a lump under the nipple. She is concerned she may have breast cancer.
HPI	She has no family history of breast cancer. She does not perform self–breast examinations, and has never had a mammogram. No other lumps in the breast axilla.
PE	VS: normal. PE: **serosanguineous discharge** from left nipple **and small cystic** swelling beneath areola; **no nipple retraction;** no other breast lumps or axillary lymphadenopathy; right breast normal.
Labs	CBC/Lytes normal.
Imaging	Mammograms show scattered microcalcifications throughout the left breast.
Micro Pathology	Cytology of nipple discharge is sent (not reliable for cancer diagnosis)

case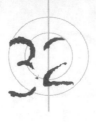

Bloody Breast Discharge

Pathogenesis

Intraductal papilloma is a benign tumor involving the epithelial lining of lactiferous ducts, and is **the most common cause of unilateral blood-stained discharge from the nipple.** The condition is **rare before the age of 25** and usually occurs in women between the **ages of 35 and 50.** Spontaneous clear, watery, or serosanguineous nipple discharge from a single duct has less than a 7% chance of being malignant.

Management

Microdochectomy (excision of duct) is the preferred treatment; however, if the duct of origin of nipple bleeding cannot be identified or when bleeding is occurring from many ducts, a ductogram may be done. If inconclusive, then consider **cone excision** of the major duct system.

Breakout Point

- The most common cause of unilateral bloody discharge from the nipple is intraductal papilloma.
- Gross bloody discharge: one third of cases malignant cause, two thirds of cases benign cause.

■ TABLE 32-1 AGE AND BREAST CANCER INCIDENCE

Age	Risk
≤ 39	1 in 235
40–59	1 in 25
60–79	1 in 15
Lifetime risk	1 in 8

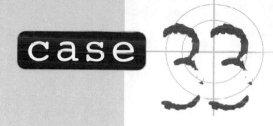

ID/CC A 65-year-old woman presents with a new **breast** lump on self-examination, and newly **inverted nipple**.

HPI She has no breast pain or discharge. No family history of breast or ovarian cancer.

PE VS: normal. PE: 2.5-cm, nonmobile, nontender mass felt in the **upper outer quadrant** (most common site of lesions) of the right breast. Inverted right nipple, but not left nipple. No nipple discharge. Right **axillary lymphadenopathy**. No hepatomegaly or bone pain. No neurologic dysfunction.

Labs CBC/Lytes normal. LFTs normal (may increase with liver metastasis). Alkaline phosphatase normal (increases with bone metastasis). Tumor markers are not used for cancer diagnosis.

Imaging Mammogram showed ill-defined mass in the right breast with multiple pleomorphic linear and branching microcalcifications. Ultrasound showed a hypoechoic mass in the upper outer quadrant of the right breast.

Micro Pathology Estrogen receptor (ER)–staining was strongly positive. Progesterone receptor (PR)–staining was positive. HER2-neu staining was negative.

GYNECOLOGIC ONCOLOGY

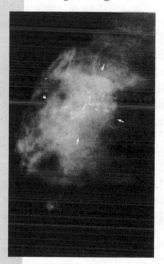

Figure 33-1. Mammogram showing breast mass with calcifications.

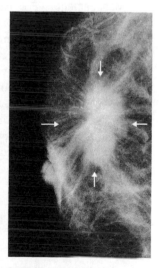

Figure 33-2. Mammogram showing breast mass causing architectural distortion.

case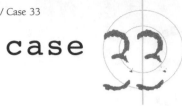

Breast Cancer

Pathogenesis

Risk factors for breast cancer include a positive **family history** (but only 10% of patients with breast cancer have positive family history), **early menarche, late menopause, late first pregnancy, nulliparity,** hormonal replacement therapy, obesity, radiation exposure (e.g., previous radiation treatment to the chest for lymphoma), high-fat diet, geographic location (North America and Western Europe), atypical hyperplasia of the breast, and breast cancer in the opposite breast. The association between oral contraception use and breast cancer risk is inconclusive. Women with mutations of **tumor suppressor genes BRCA-1 or BRCA-2** are at increased risk of developing breast cancer; BRCA-1 is also associated with ovarian cancer. Breastfeeding is protective. Inflammatory breast cancer shows angiolymphatic spread and has an aggressive course with early, widespread metastases.

Management

For early breast cancer, breast-conserving surgery (LUMPECTOMY) **with radiation is equivalent to mastectomy in cure rate.** Staging of axillary nodes is most commonly done with sentinel node biopsy; if positive, axillary dissection is done. **Adjuvant chemotherapy** is aimed at preventing distant metastases in larger tumors and in advanced disease. For HER2/neu-positive tumors, **Herceptin** is added to the chemotherapy regimen. **Tamoxifen** is given for ER- or PR-positive tumors.

Breakout Point

- New nipple retraction, older age, and axillary lymphadenopathy give this case away, even before the mammogram and biopsy.

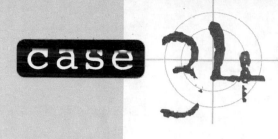

case 24

ID/CC	A 49-year-old premenopausal woman presents with **abnormal Pap smear on routine screening.**
HPI	The patient reports no abnormal vaginal bleeding or discharge. She has smoked 2 packs of cigarettes a day since age 22. Her first pregnancy was at 15 years of age. History of *Chlamydia* infection.
PE	VS: normal. Pelvic examination reveals normal-sized uterus; a small friable lesion is seen on the cervix. No palpable inguinal lymphadenopathy.
Labs	CBC: normal. UA: normal.
Imaging	Normal chest X-ray and pelvic CT.
Gross Pathology	Punch biopsy is performed. (If no cervical lesion is seen on examination, colposcopy with directed biopsy is necessary for diagnosis. If colposcopy is non-diagnostic, conization should be done).
Micro Pathology	Pap smear showed atypical squamous cells.

case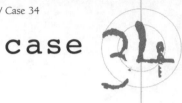

Cervical Cancer

Pathogenesis

Human papillomavirus (subtypes 16, 18, 31) implicated in the pathogenesis of cervical cancer is found in the transformation zone, at the junction of the squamous and columnar epithelia (SQUAMOCOLUMNAR JUNCTION). There is also a **synergistic association between HIV and HPV;** women infected with both viruses are at an even higher risk for cervical cancer. The most common variety is **squamous cell;** less common is adenocarcinoma. **Multiple male sexual partners, early onset of sexual activity, HPV or other sexually transmitted diseases,** and **smoking** are risk factors for developing cervical cancer.

Management

Pap smear is the gold standard for screening and should be initiated with the onset of sexual activity. **Colposcopy** and **biopsy** is performed for diagnosis. Cervical cancer is **staged clinically** by PE, chest X-ray, cystoscopy, IV pyelogram, and proctoscopy (the last three are often replaced by CT scan or MRI). For **carcinoma in situ,** conization with surveillance is indicated for women who wish to bear children; hysterectomy is warranted if they have completed childbirth.

Breakout Point

Cervical cancer HPV subtypes:

- 16, 18, 31. (Types 6 and 11 predispose to condylomas.)
- Symptoms: abnormal vaginal bleeding, postcoital bleeding, vaginal discharge. But more patients are now diagnosed via screening Pap smear, without symptoms.
- Mean age of diagnosis is 47.

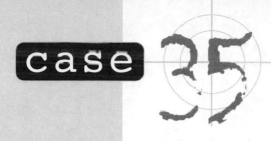

case 25

ID/CC A 40-year-old woman presents with increasing **shortness of breath** (DYSPNEA) and **blood-tinged sputum** (HEMOPTYSIS; due to pulmonary metastases). She also complains of severe **nausea**, occasional vomiting, and **intermittent vaginal bleeding.**

HPI The patient had a dilation and vacuum aspiration (SUCTION CURETTAGE) 6 months ago for a **hydatidiform mole.** She has not kept her scheduled follow-up visits for surveillance β-hCG levels and CXRs.

PE VS: normal. PE: **pallor;** scattered rales in lungs; no abdominal masses; **increase in size of uterus;** no adnexal masses; speculum examination reveals **bluish-red vascular tumor.**

Labs CBC: mild anemia. LFTs: alkaline phosphatase normal. TFTs: normal. UA: normal. **Elevated serum and urinary hCG levels.**

Imaging **CXR and chest CT: multiple nodules** (CANNONBALL METASTASES). **Pelvic ultrasound: increased size of uterus,** with solid echogenic material in the myometrium.

Gross Pathology Tumor with **red, granulated appearance** with specific areas of central necrosis and hemorrhage.

Micro Pathology Confirms **choriocarcinoma.** Consists of mixed **syncytiotrophoblastic and cytotrophoblastic** tissue with multiple abnormal mitoses, multinucleated giant cells, and extensive areas of necrosis and hemorrhage. No villi are noted.

case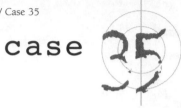

Hydatidiform Mole/Choriocarcinoma

Pathogenesis

Choriocarcinoma is a **highly anaplastic gestational trophoblastic malignancy** (the spectrum of the disease also includes hydatidiform mole and invasive mole) that involves the proliferation of trophoblast cells but **does not contain villi.** Levels of hCG should return to normal by 12 weeks after molar pregnancy evacuation; if the level plateaus or rises, or if it increases in the absence of pregnancy after having returned to normal, choriocarcinoma should be strongly suspected. It invades locally and disseminates early hematogenously; the **most common sites of spread are the lungs and vagina.** Sometimes the first signs of choriocarcinoma are metastases to the external genitalia, vagina, or rectum.

Epidemiology

Most commonly develops after evacuation of a hydatidiform mole, although may also occur after normal pregnancies, ectopic pregnancies, miscarriages, or therapeutic abortions. Factors associated with poor prognosis are hCG levels >40,000, disease >4 months' duration, brain/liver metastases, failure of prior chemotherapy, and antecedent term pregnancy (see Table 35-1 for details).

Management

Chemotherapy may consist of single therapy or combination therapy. Radiotherapy may be employed in disease involving brain or liver metastases.

Complications

Complications include CNS, liver, and kidney metastases.

Breakout Point

> FIGO staging for gestational trophoblastic neoplasia is as follows. Stage I = confined to uterus, stage II = metastasis to vagina or pelvis, stage III = metastasis to lung, stage IV = other distant metastases.

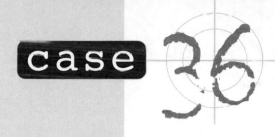
ID/CC   A 54-year-old postmenopausal woman is referred to the surgical clinic after a mammogram detected a new **cluster of microcalcifications** in the right breast.

HPI   The patient has faithfully had annual mammograms, and denies breast pain or discharge. She is otherwise well, and has never received hormonal replacement therapy. Her **sister had breast cancer** 1 year ago, and is doing well after treatment.

PE   VS: normal. Examination shows symmetric breasts without skin erythema or nipple inversion. There is no palpable breast mass, or cervical/supraclavicular/axillary lymphadenopathy.

Labs   Not applicable.

Imaging   Mammogram findings as above; the patient has dense breasts. Breast ultrasound does not show a clear right breast mass.

Gross Pathology   Needle localization biopsy of the microcalcifications shows ductal carcinoma in situ (DCIS), ER (estrogen receptor) and PR (progesterone receptor) positive.

GYNECOLOGIC ONCOLOGY

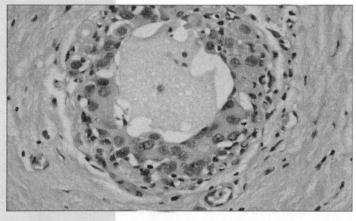

Figure 36-1. Photomicrograph of ductal carcinoma in situ. The abnormal cells do not cross the ductal basement membrane, therefore making this a preinvasive lesion.

case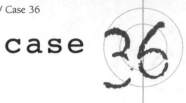

Ductal Carcinoma in Situ

Pathogenesis

DCIS, (ductal carcinoma in situ) is the collection of preinvasive malignant epithelial cells. Risk factors for DCIS are similar to those for invasive breast cancer, and include **family history, early menarche, late menopause, late first pregnancy, nulliparity,** hormonal replacement therapy, and obesity. 80% of DCIS cases are detected via screening mammograms in asymptomatic patients.

Management

Surgical complete excision of the lesion is required (i.e., **lumpectomy**); repeat surgeries may be necessary to achieve negative margins. (Even if biopsy shows DCIS, it is possible that, because of sampling error, another part of the lesion may contain invasive cancer.) Standard adjuvant treatment includes breast irradiation, and hormonal therapy (e.g., tamoxifen) if the tumor is ER or PR positive. Mastectomy is an alternative surgical treatment, though most patients prefer breast-conserving surgery if it is possible. Chemotherapy is not indicated for DCIS.

Breakout Point

- If cure is not achieved, recurrence may be in the form of DCIS (50%) or invasive breast cancer (50%).

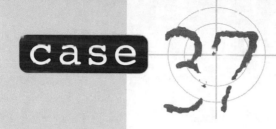

case 37

ID/CC	A 59-year-old woman presents with vague abdominal symptoms (including **lower abdominal pressure and bloating**) for several months, not alleviated by over-the-counter medication.
HPI	She also reports **increased abdominal girth**, occasional diarrhea alternating with constipation, early satiety with 30-lb **weight loss**, and increased shortness of breath over 1 month.
PE	VS: normal. PE: no acute distress; abdomen nontender; with ascites present; **mass felt** in left iliac fossa (in postmenopausal women, regarded as **malignant until proven otherwise**); no peritoneal signs; pelvic examination confirms **left fixed, nontender, irregular solid adnexal mass;** cervix normal; rectal examination normal. Significantly decreased breath sounds in the lower half of left lung.
Labs	CBC/Lytes: normal. **CA-125 elevated.** LFTs. normal. Blood glucose normal. UA: normal.
Imaging	CXR: left-sided pleural effusion. CT/US, pelvis: cystic mass 6 cm in diameter with solid areas in the left ovary; omental caking; ascites.
Micro Pathology	Thoracentesis and paracentesis both show malignant cells.

GYNECOLOGIC ONCOLOGY

case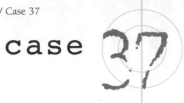

Ovarian Cancer

Pathogenesis

Risk factors include **family history** of ovarian cancer, **nulligravity, delayed childbirth, early menarche,** and **late age at menopause.** Women with **breast cancer** have a twofold increase in ovarian cancer. **Oral contraception, multiparity, breastfeeding, and tubal ligation** are **protective.** Because of the nonspecific symptoms, ovarian carcinoma often attains considerable size before it is detected; nearly 75% of cases have **metastases at diagnosis.** Of all ovarian cancers, **90% are epithelial in origin.** Of these, the most common variety is **serous cystadenocarcinoma** (may also be mucinous); other types include solid endometrioid carcinomas and Brenner tumors. 20% of ovarian cancers are derived from the germ cell of the ovary (e.g., teratomas, dysgerminomas); 10% originate from the ovarian stroma (e.g., fibromas, granulosa-theca cell tumors). Ovarian carcinoma spreads **lymphatically** to the regional nodes, **directly** through peritoneal seeding, and **hematogenously** to the liver, bone, and lungs. Carcinoma of the ovary is not always primary; secondary ovarian malignancy them stomach cancer metastasis is called Krukenberg tumor.

Management

Total abdominal hysterectomy with **bilateral salpingo-oophorectomy,** omentectomy, and lymphadenectomy if the tumor is in its early stages. For advanced disease, there is a survival advantage to surgically **debulking** of the tumor. Adjuvant therapy consists of **chemotherapy.**

Breakout Point

- CA-125 is not used for diagnosis of ovarian cancer, but is followed serially to assess treatment efficacy and disease recurrence.
- Associated with BRCA1 and BRCA2 mutations.

■ TABLE 37-1 FIGO (SURGICAL) STAGING FOR OVARIAN CANCER

Stage	Description
1	Tumor confined to one or both ovaries (including cases with capsules ruptured and positive peritoneal cytology)
2	Pelvic extension (including fallopian tubes, uterus, other pelvic structures)
3	Peritoneal implants (including **surface** implants on liver, bowel, omentum) or positive nodes
4	Distant metastases (including parenchymal lesions in liver)

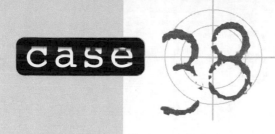

case 28

ID/CC A 62-year-old postmenopausal woman presents with **vaginal bleeding.**

HPI She reports bleeding with large clots for 7 days, requiring several pads a day, and a 20-lb **weight loss** over the past 3 months. No pelvic pain or rectal/ urinary symptoms. Never been pregnant. Pap smear 2 years ago was normal.

PE VS: normal. PE: **obese,** pale, and ill-looking; atrophic vulva; speculum examination reveals old blood in cervical canal and vagina; uterus **enlarged but mobile; no adnexal swelling;** cervix patulous; clot seen protruding from os. Rectovaginal examination reveals tumor did not extend into the rectum. Uterine cavity D&C confirmed a wide, expanded cavity; **necrotic tumor obtained from all surfaces; curettage provoked bleeding.**

Labs CBC: **normocytic, normochromic anemia** (blood loss).

Imaging Transvaginal ultrasound reveals enlarged uterus and thickened endometrium. Pelvic CT shows an irregular uterine mass without abnormal lymphadenopathy.

Micro Pathology Pap smear reveals atrophic tissue.

Gross Pathology Endocervical curettage reveals **no tumor;** endometrial curettage is performed.

case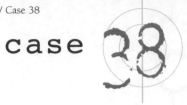

Postmenopausal Bleeding (Uterine Cancer)

Pathogenesis

Risk factors include **unopposed estrogen use, tamoxifen, obesity, nulliparity, chronic anovulation,** diabetes, hypertension, **early menarche, and family history.** **Smoking** (by inducing hepatic metabolism of estrogens), physical activity, and oral contraceptives are **protective.** The tumor is spread primarily by direct extension to the cervix and myometrium through the fallopian tubes to the peritoneum and via the lymphatics to the pelvic and para-aortic lymph nodes. Most common histology is adenocarcinoma (80%).

Management

Any woman with postmenopausal bleeding should be worked up with a Pap smear, endocervical curettage, and endometrial biopsy. Because FIGO staging for uterine cancer is surgery based, the primary treatment modality is **total abdominal hysterectomy and bilateral salpingo-oophorectomy.** For **stage I disease,** surgery is usually sufficient; postoperative radiation therapy may also be given. **Stage II, III, and IVA disease** would require postoperative chemotherapy and radiation. Patients with distant metastasis **(stage IVB)** are usually treated with chemotherapy only; surgery and radiation treatment may be needed for palliation.

■ **TABLE 38-1 FIGO (SURGICAL) STAGING OF ENDOMETRIAL CANCER**

Stage	Description
0	Carcinoma in situ
I	Tumor confined to corpus uteri. 1A: confined to endometrium. 1B: invades up to half the thickness of myometrium. 1C: more than half the thickness of myometrium
2	Tumor invades the cervix, but is still confined to the uterus
3A	Tumor involves uterine serosa and/or adnexa. Or positive peritoneal washings
3B	Vaginal involvement
3C	Positive pelvic or para-aortic nodes
4A	Local invasion of bladder or bowel
4B	Distant metastasis

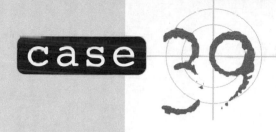

case 39

ID/CC	A 38-year-old G3P3 woman presents with **heavy, prolonged menstrual bleeding** for several years.
HPI	She also reports worsening **pelvic pressure** and **dysmenorrhea**. She is not interested in future child-bearing.
PE	VS: normal. Speculum examination demonstrates a normal cervix without lesions. The uterus is **enlarged to approximately 14 cm** on bimanual examination, with **multiple firm nodularities**. Several are mobile on examination. Adnexa are nonpalpable; no leg edema.
Labs	Hemoglobin 9.2 g/dL; serum iron 12 ng/mL (low); ferritin 8 ng/mL (low). PT/PTT/INR normal.
Imaging	Pelvic ultrasound shows uterus with **multiple submucosal, intramural, and subserosal masses,** the largest measuring 6 cm.
Gross Pathology	Endometrial biopsy shows benign tissue without hyperplasia.
Micro Pathology	Pap smear is negative. Peripheral blood smear shows **hypochromic, microcytic anemia** (chronic iron deficiency anemia due to increased bleeding).

GYNECOLOGIC ONCOLOGY

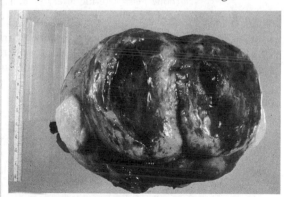

Figure 39-1. This uterine module is well circumscribed, with a bulging, white, firm, whorled cut surface. The mass is soft, hemorrhagic fleshy.

case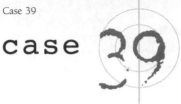

Uterine Fibroids

Pathogenesis

Uterine fibroids (leiomyomas) are **benign estrogen-dependent tumors** that originate from **smooth muscle cells**. Uterine fibroids may be **subserosal** (on the serosal side of the uterine wall), **intramural** (located in the myometrium, most common type), or **submucosal** (protruding toward the uterine cavity), and can be single or multiple. Fibroids can range in size from microscopic to >20 cm. Symptomatology varies depending on the sizes and locations of fibroids, with submucosal leiomyomas most likely to cause irregular bleeding. These tumors are **responsive to sex steroid hormones** and typically regress after menopause.

Management

Endometrial biopsy should be performed to rule out malignancy or hyperplasia; Pap smear should also be performed. Expectant management is recommended for asymptomatic women. For women who have completed childbearing, **hysterectomy** can be offered as **definitive surgical management**. **Myomectomy** can be considered in symptomatic patients who desire uterine preservation. Medical therapy such as hormonal contraception can assist with menorrhagia. GnRH-agonists can decrease fibroid size and improve symptoms; however, long-term use is limited by side effects (bone loss). Uterine artery embolization is emerging as a newer, minimally invasive alternative for select patients.

Complications

Patients may experience **urinary frequency, constipation, and hydronephrosis** due to compression of pelvic structures. Other reproductive complications such as infertility, recurrent pregnancy loss, and preterm labor may occur.

Breakout Point

- Menorrhagia is the most common type of abnormal uterine bleeding associated with uterine fibroids.
- African American women are 2–3 times more likely to have fibroids than women of other racial groups.
- Malignant transformation to leiomyosarcoma occurs rarely in <1% of cases.
- Fibroids are the most common tumors affecting women and the most common surgical indication for hysterectomy.

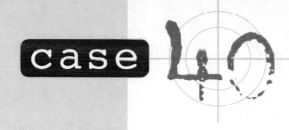

case 40

ID/CC   A 53-year-old woman presents with **postcoital bleeding** and **malodorous vaginal discharge.**

HPI   She had a **history of cervical cancer,** treated 10 years ago with radical hysterectomy; no sign of recurrence and deemed cured.

PE   VS: normal. PE: Speculum examination reveals a 1.5-cm **mass in the upper third of vagina,** on the posterior wall. This lesion bleeds easily. Cervix was previously surgically removed. Rectovaginal examination reveals tumor does not extend into the rectum; there is no parametrial thickening.

Labs   CBC/Lytes: normal.

Imaging   CXR normal.

Gross Pathology   Biopsy of the vaginal lesion is sent.

case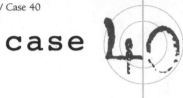

Vaginal Cancer

Pathogenesis

Risk factors for vaginal cancer and vaginal intraepithelial neoplasia (VAIN) are similar to cervical cancer, and include **multiple sexual partners, early age of first intercourse, HPV 16/18, and smoking.** Women exposed to **diethylstilbestrol (DES) in utero** can develop **clear-cell adenocarcinoma of the vagina,** usually before age 30. VAIN is defined by neoplastic cells without invasion, and is categorized into VAIN I, II, and III based on the cells involving one third, two thirds, or more than two thirds of the epithelium. Vaginal carcinoma in situ is included under VAIN III. Invasive vaginal cancer spreads by **direct** extension or by **lymphatic** and **hematologic** spread.

Management

Biopsy is necessary to establish diagnosis. Cystoscopy and proctoscopy are done for staging, and to rule out extension of tumor into the rectum or bladder. Lymph node status is not part of staging. If VAIN is diagnosed, **colposcopy and biopsy** must be performed to rule out invasive disease. VAIN treatment options include surgical excision, CO_2 laser ablation, topical fluorouracil, and radiation therapy. Stage I vaginal cancer less than 2 cm in the upper vagina can be treated with surgery (radical hysterectomy, upper vaginectomy, and pelvic lymphadenectomy). Larger stage I lesions, and stage II to IV disease, are treated with radiation, often combined with concurrent chemotherapy.

Breakout Point

- Mean age at diagnosis is 60.
- The majority of vaginal malignancies are metastases rather than primary vaginal cancer.
- Most common histology is squamous cell carcinoma (83%), followed by adenocarcinoma (9%), sarcoma (3%), and melanoma (3%).
- Most common location is the posterior wall of the upper third of vagina.

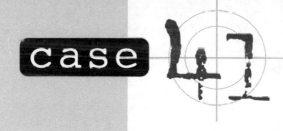

case 47

ID/CC	A **63-year-old** woman complains of an ulcer on her **left labia majora** that has persisted for several months.
HPI	The patient has had **vulvar pruritus** for several months, which she has been unsuccessfully treating with various creams. For the past 2 days, she has also noticed some **bleeding** and staining of her undergarments.
PE	VS: normal. PE: no abdominal masses and no inguinal lymphadenopathy. Vulva shows 2.5-cm **ulcerating lesion** on posterior aspect of right labia majora with rolled, **indurated edges;** easy bleeding; and surrounding hypopigmentation; vaginal examination reveals atrophic mucosal surface; cervix normal; no pelvic masses; rectal examination reveals normal sphincter tone with no masses.
Labs	CBC/lytes: normal. FSH and LH elevated (because of menopause)
Imaging	CXR: unfolded aortic knob; mild cardiomegaly; no infiltrates; no signs of metastatic disease. IVP: normal.
Gross Pathology	Excisional biopsy of vulvar lesion is performed.

GYNECOLOGIC ONCOLOGY

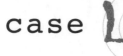 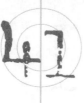

case 41

Vulvar Cancer

Pathogenesis

Vulvar intraepithelial neoplasia (VIN) stages I, II, and III are considered premalignant conditions that may progress to invasive vulvar carcinoma. Risk factors include **human papillomavirus subtypes 16, 18, and 31** smoking; vulvar dystrophy (e.g., lichen sclerosis); immunodeficiency; history of cervical cancer; and Northern European descent. As in cervical cancer, VIN precedes the development of invasive carcinoma by many years. Vulvar carcinoma may be ulcerating or fungating (EXOPHYTIC), as well as macular or papular; fungating lesions or ulcers are not always seen. Tumors invade by **local extension** and by **lymphatic spread.**

Management

Lesions of the vulva that look suspicious should be biopsied. Toluidine blue and colposcopy may help when selecting sites for biopsy. If locally advanced disease suspected IV pyelogram will rule out kidney/ureteral disease and will detect possible local GU invasion, and sigmoidoscopy can rule out rectal invasion. **Vulvar intraepithelial neoplasia** may be treated by skinning vulvectomy, **wide local excision,** or laser. For vulvar cancer, **surgical resection** is the mainstay of treatment for stage I to stage III disease; inguinofemoral nodal dissection is usually done. Adjuvant radiation is indicated for patients with positive nodes or positive/close surgical margins. Stage IV disease may require pelvic exenteration (surgical removal of bladder, urethra, vagina, cervix, uterus, fallopian tubes, ovaries, rectum, anus, and vulva) and/or concurrent chemoradiation.

Breakout Point

- Mean age at diagnosis is 65.
- Most common histologic type is squamous cell >90%). Other histologies include melanoma (5%), basal cell carcinoma (2%), and sarcoma (2%).
- Most commonly on labia majora. Labia minora, clitoris, perineum, and mons are less common.

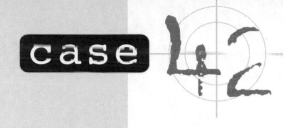

case 42

ID/CC A 32-year-old G2P0010 at 37 weeks presents with **nausea and vomiting.**

HPI The nausea and vomiting developed over the last few hours, along with **mild right upper quadrant pain.** Her antepartum course has been benign, although she has developed intense thirst over the last day.

PE VS: Afebrile, stable. Jaundiced woman. Abdomen significant for right upper quadrant tenderness, no rebound or guarding. Uterus measures size equaling dates.

Labs ALT 102, AST 110, albumin 4.6; WBC 18, Hct 38, Plts 100K, INR 2.0; glucose 86, conjugated bilirubin 12, Cr 1.2; 1+ pro on UA.

Imaging Right upper quadrant ultrasound reveals a hyperechoic liver, patent portal vessels, and a normal gallbladder with a small amount of sludging.

Gross Pathology Liver biopsy reveals microvesicular fatty infiltration of hepatocytes.

case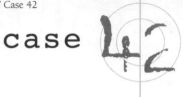

Acute Fatty Liver of Pregnancy

Pathogenesis

Acute fatty liver of pregnancy (AFLP), along with Reye syndrome, are diseases of **microvesicular fatty infiltration.** Pathogenesis is unclear, although β-oxidation deficiency has been implicated in some cases.

Management

The diagnosis of acute fatty liver of pregnancy is made clinically. **Liver biopsy** is the gold standard for diagnosis, but is invasive and can be dangerous in cases of concurrent coagulopathy. Hospitalization and delivery is indicated.

Complications

Cerebral edema, liver and renal failure, hypoglycemia, GI hemorrhage, coagulopathy, infections, fetal death, PPH, maternal mortality.

Breakout Point

- AFLP is considered a medical emergency, for which delivery is recommended for recovery.
- Severe AFLP can be indistinguishable from preeclampsia and HELLP syndrome.
- Liver biopsy is confirmatory, but diagnosis is usually based on clinical and laboratory criteria rather than histologic criteria because timely management is crucial.

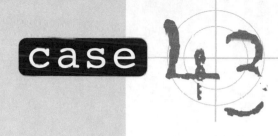

case 43

ID/CC	A **38-year-old** G4P4004 woman **suddenly develops laborious breathing** and light-headedness **following a vaginal delivery.**
HPI	The patient is a **multigravida** who underwent complicated delivery with prolonged second stage because of a **large fetus (9 lbs 8 oz).** Her falling BP and tachycardia are unresponsive to fluid resuscitation.
PE	VS: tachycardia (HR 130); hypotension (BP 80/50); tachypnea (RR 26). PE: **cold, clammy skin; dyspneic, cyanotic, and comatose;** weak, thready pulse; generalized tonic-clonic **convulsions** begin a few minutes after delivery. Ultimately, cardiopulmonary arrest ensues and the patient expires despite attempts to revive her.
Labs	CBC: **thrombocytopenia. Decreased fibrinogen; prolonged bleeding time and PT/PTT; elevated fibrin split products** (due to DIC) and D-dimer.
Imaging	CXR: severe **pulmonary edema.**
Gross Pathology	Fetal debris evident within the pulmonary vasculature.
Micro Pathology	Fetal squamous cells evident in the maternal pulmonary circulation, obstructing capillaries.

■ **TABLE 43-1 SIGNS AND SYMPTOMS NOTED IN PATIENTS WITH THIS CONDITION**

Sign or Symptom	No. Patients	%
Hypotension	43	100
Fetal distress	30	100
Pulmonary edema or adult respiratory distress syndrome	28	93
Cardiopulmonary arrest	40	87
Cyanosis	38	83
Coagulopathy	38	83
Dyspnea	22	49
Seizure	22	48
Uterine atony	11	23
Bronchospasm	7	15
Transient hypertension	5	11
Cough	3	7
Headache	3	7
Chest Pain	1	2

case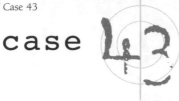

Amniotic Fluid Embolism

Pathogenesis

The pathophysiology of amniotic fluid embolism is not well understood. Particulate matter, such as fetal squamous cells, vernix, or amniotic fluid, gains access to the maternal circulation through lacerations in the placental membrane and rupture of uteroplacental veins, likely triggering an anaphylactic reaction to fetal antigens or activation of the complement cascade. This in turn leads to severe, acute **pulmonary hypertension and hypoxia.** If she survives this initial insult, the second phase of the disorder results in a hemorrhagic phase, including **massive hemorrhage with DIC.** **Diagnosis is clinical** because the presence of squamous cells in maternal blood is not enough to confirm a diagnosis of amniotic fluid embolism.

Epidemiology

Amniotic fluid embolism is a rare obstetric complication occurring in 1 per 50,000 deliveries (after vaginal delivery, abortion, or cesarean section). If it occurs in the delivery period, it may be associated with **abruptio placentae** and fetal death. Predisposing factors include **older age,** uterine rupture, and twin pregnancy with uterine overdistention.

Management

If the patient survives initial resuscitation, she should be admitted to the ICU for close hemodynamic monitoring, oxygen, ventilatory support, treatment of acute heart failure, and continued treatment of DIC.

Complications

Death results in 80% of cases. Neurologic damage due to hypoxia is a true concern in patients who survive amniotic fluid embolism (approximately 50%).

Breakout Point

- Amniotic fluid embolism (AFE) is a rare, but deadly, obstetrical complication with mortality reportedly as high as 80%.
- Pathophysiology is poorly understood; however, it is likely the result of an anaphylactic reaction to fetal antigens.
- Initial signs of AFE include extreme hypotension, tachycardia, and hypoxemia.

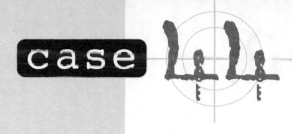

case

ID/CC	A 25-year-old **G1P0** has been in active labor for over 8 hours. During the last 2 hours her cervix has **stopped dilating**, at 8 cm, and her **contractions have become weaker and less frequent**.
HPI	The patient is 39 weeks and 2 days past her LMP (last menstrual period). Last ultrasound examination at 36 weeks showed that the fetus was **not in breech position. Rupture of membranes** was approximately 4 hours ago.
PE	VS: maternal—normal; fetal—HR 150s, **no signs of distress** on heart monitor. Mother appears tired but otherwise well. A sterile vaginal examination shows that the cervix remains dilated to at 8 cm and the fetal head can be felt in the **occiput posterior position** (important to verify the position of the baby and ensure that malpresentation (breech, compound, etc.) is not causing prolonged labor).

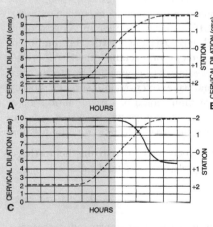

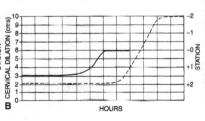

Figure 44-1. Examples of different arrest disorders. **(A)** Prolonged latent phase (change into the active phase is arrested). **(B)** Arrest of dilation, in which cervix achieves 6 cm of dilation but then does not change for 2 hours. **(C)** Arrest of descent, in which the fetal head moves from a −2 station to a 0 to −1 station, but then makes no further progress.

OBSTETRICS

case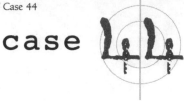

Arrested Labor

Pathogenesis

There are three stages of labor: time from onset of labor to complete cervical dilation (first stage), to delivery of fetus (second stage), to delivery of placenta (third stage). The first stage is further divided into latent phase (mild and infrequent contractions with cervical dilation <1 cm/hr) and active phase (intense and regular contractions with cervical dilation >1 cm/hr). Protraction of labor is defined as slower-than-normal labor progress, whereas arrested labor refers to cessation of progress. Protraction or arrested labor can be due abnormalities of the cervix, uterus, maternal pelvis, or fetus. Causes include **hypocontractile uterus** (most common cause during the first stage of labor), **epidural anesthesia,** and **cephalopelvic discordance** (disproportion between size of the fetus relative to the mother). Positions other than occiput anterior (such as **occiput posterior** or **transverse** positions) can also cause protracted or arrested labor.

Management

The choice between medical management versus a cesarean section depends on **degree of uterine activity, length and progression of ongoing labor, CPD, fetal presentation, and fetal health status.** Delays during the first stage can be managed with **amniotomy** and **oxytocin,** and an intrauterine pressure (**IUP**) catheter to monitor contractions. During the second stage, **assistance with fetal rotation or extraction with forceps or vacuum** can be performed. Delivery of the placenta can be augmented by **uterine massage, oxytocin, manual extraction, and surgery,** if necessary. A **cesarean section** should be carried out as soon as possible if it is felt that the mother will be unable to deliver on her own, or if the maternal or fetal health is in question.

Complications

Chorioamnionitis, increased postpartum hemorrhage, hysterectomy, cord prolapse, and fetal demise.

Breakout Point

- Arrested labor is the most common cause of unplanned cesarean sections.
- About 95% of occiput posterior positions spontaneously revert to the anterior position (more conducive to vaginal birth).

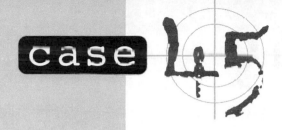
ID/CC A 32-year-old G2P1 presents for routine prenatal visit at 36 weeks gestation.

HPI The patient has received routine prenatal care and has had an uncomplicated pregnancy. No leaking fluid, vaginal bleeding, or contractions. Active fetal movements have been noted.

PE VS: normal. Fundal height: 34 cm. Fetal heart rate is 155, and is auscultated near the uterine fundus. **Leopold maneuvers** (to ascertain fetal position) reveal a firm mass in the right upper quadrant; **presenting part is soft** and not engaged in the maternal pelvis.

Labs Not applicable.

Imaging Transabdominal ultrasound reveals the fetus to be in frank breech presentation with the back at the maternal left.

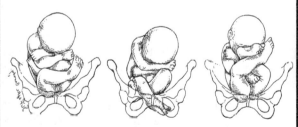

Figure 45-1. Frank, incomplete, and complete breech presentations.

OBSTETRICS

case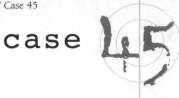

Breech Presentation

Pathogenesis

Up to 30% of fetuses prior to 32 weeks gestation are breech (i.e., buttock first); at term, only 4% remain so. Factors predisposing to breech presentation at term include fetal anomalies (hydrocephalus, anencephaly, autosomal trisomy), uterine anomalies (septate or bicornuate uterus), polyhydramnios, obstruction by placenta previa or leiomyomata, or high parity with lax abdominal/uterine musculature. **Frank breech** is most common (hips flexed, knees extended; 60–65%), followed by **incomplete** (hips incompletely flexed, extremity presenting; 25–35%), and finally **complete** (hips and knees both flexed; 5%).

Management

In 2001, the American College of Obstetricians and Gynecologists officially advised **cesarean delivery** for all singleton breech fetuses. This restriction does not apply to patients presenting in advanced labor in whom delivery is imminent, or to a breech-presenting second twin. The patient may choose an attempted **external cephalic version** (ECV) first. If successful, labor may then be induced. ECV carries a poorly defined risk of fetal bradycardia and placental abruption, either of which may necessitate emergent cesarean delivery. Contraindications to attempting ECV include rupture of membranes, engaged presenting part, and active labor.

Complications

Fetuses delivered vaginally from the breech presentation are at higher risk for perinatal morbidity. The head does not spend time in the pelvis and is thus not molded, making head entrapment with subsequent trauma a significant risk. Traction or tight grasping of fetal parts other than the bony pelvis can damage soft tissues. There is also significant risk of cord prolapse, leading to asphyxia.

Breakout Point

- 4% of fetuses at term are in breech presentation.
- Associated with fetal anomalies, uterine anomalies, and polyhydramnios.
- Vaginal delivery not advised because of risk for birth trauma and asphyxia.

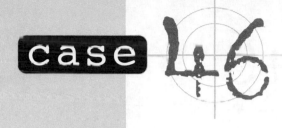

ID/CC	A 19-year-old G3P0020, at approximately 38 weeks, complains of new-onset **abdominal pain** with **fever** and chills.
HPI	She has had no prenatal care. Her dating is based on an uncertain last menstrual period. She thought she felt a gush of fluid 2 days ago, but is not sure.
PE	VS: febrile (102.5°F/39.0°C); HR 120, normal BP. PE: uncomfortable. Abdomen reveals a term gravid uterus, but significant **uterine tenderness.** Pelvic examination shows **thick, yellowish-green cervical discharge.** There is **foul-smelling** fluid in the vagina that is **fern-test and nitrazine-test positive.** Vaginal examination reveals a 5-cm dilated cervix. Fetal heart monitoring demonstrated fetal tachycardia (HR 160) with loss of variability and no decelerations.
Labs	CBC: anemia; leukocytosis (23,000) with left shift (90% neutrophils, 2% bandemia). UA/Lytes: normal.
Imaging	US: scant amniotic fluid; no fetal abnormalities except for tachycardia. Fetal weight and measurements are within 3 weeks of estimated gestational age.
Gross Pathology	None.
Micro Pathology	Amniotic fluid culture yields mixed flora and group B streptococcus.

OBSTETRICS

case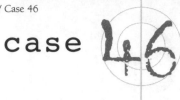

Chorioamnionitis

Pathogenesis

Chorioamnionitis, or **infection of the fetal membranes and amniotic fluid,** is most frequently caused by ascending infections and hematogenous spread. The most common causative organisms are anaerobes, group B *Streptococcus*, and *E. coli*. Risk factors include nulliparity, prolonged rupture of membranes (PROM) (>18 hours), prolonged labor, preexisting infections, and multiple digital vaginal examinations.

Epidemiology

Chorioamnionitis complicates about 1% of all deliveries. In PROM >18 hours, there is a significantly higher incidence of chorioamnionitis; in preterm PROM, the incidence may reach 40%.

Management

The diagnosis is made with maternal fever and at least two of the following: maternal tachycardia, maternal leukocytosis, fundal tenderness, fetal tachycardia, and foul-smelling amniotic fluid. Gold standard for diagnosis is **amniotic fluid culture,** which may be done in the setting of prematurity. **Antibiotic therapy** includes ampicillin, gentamicin, and clindamycin. Delivery is necessary if the diagnosis is confirmed, but method (e.g., cesarean section) should only be dictated by obstetrical concerns.

Complications

Maternal: abnormal labor progression, cesarean section, puerperal infection (endometritis, pelvic abscess, septic pelvic thrombophlebitis), postpartum hemorrhage, sepsis, DIC, renal failure, ARDS, death. Neonatal: pneumonia, sepsis, cerebral palsy, neurodevelopmental delay, death.

Breakout Point

- Chorioamnionitis is a diagnosis made with maternal fever and at least two of the following: maternal tachycardia, maternal leukocytosis, fundal tenderness, fetal tachycardia, and foul-smelling amniotic fluid.
- Broad-coverage antibiotics are needed because the cause of chorioamnionitis is often polymicrobial.

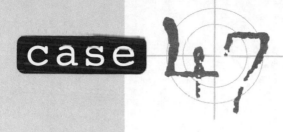

case 47

ID/CC   A 26-year-old G1P0 at 42 weeks gestation is admitted to Labor and Delivery in early labor. On admission, fetal heart rate was noted to be reassuring, in the 140s with accelerations noted, no decelerations, and moderate variability. The patient now has contractions every 3 minutes, and tracings now show **late decelerations** to 90 with almost every contraction.

HPI   The patient had spontaneous rupture of membranes with clear fluid 3 hours prior to admission. She has received routine prenatal care, and denies any complications with the pregnancy. The decelerations on the fetal heart tracing are **U shaped**, occur after the beginning of the contraction, and end after the contraction has ended. The **nadir of the deceleration is after the peak of the contraction. Minimal variability** is noted in between the contractions.

PE   VS: normal. Sterile vaginal examination: 5 cm/100/ −2 (cervix dilated to 5 cm, 100% effacement, fetus at 2 cm above the cervix). No acceleration of the heart rate is noted with **scalp stimulation** (indicates likely fetal acidosis).

Labs   Not applicable.

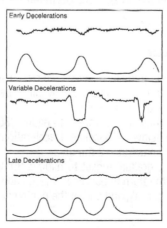

Figure 47-1. Different deceleration patterns.

case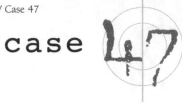

Deceleration of Fetal Heart Rate

Pathogenesis | **Early decelerations** are thought to be caused by vagal nerve activation from fetal head compression; **variable decelerations** are thought to be caused by umbilical cord compression. **Late decelerations** are due to uteroplacental insufficiency. The resultant hypoxia leads to fetal shunting of blood to vital organs (i.e., brain, heart, placenta) via constriction of peripheral arteries; the hypertension from arterial constriction activates baroreceptors, which leads to vagal stimulation of the fetal heart and lowering of the heart rate. Late decelerations are a worrisome sign and may progress to fetal bradycardia.

Management | Treatment for a nonreassuring deceleration pattern includes **supplemental O_2, change in maternal position** (which may increase blood flow to the placenta), maternal IV fluid bolus, and a sterile vaginal examination to check for an umbilical cord prolapse. Scalp stimulation is performed to rule out fetal acidosis. If the above maneuvers do not improve the fetal heart tracing, immediate delivery is necessary and a cesarean section may be indicated.

Complications | Fetal acidosis and perinatal mortality.

Breakout Point |

Differential Diagnosis

- Early decelerations: gradual (onset to nadir ≥30 seconds) decrease in fetal heart rate with return to baseline. Nadir of deceleration occurs at same time as peak of contractions.
- Variable decelerations: abrupt (onset to nadir <30 seconds) decrease in fetal heart rate below the baseline. Deceleration is ≥15 bpm lasting more than 15 seconds but <2 minutes.
- Late decelerations: gradual (onset to nadir ≥30 seconds) decrease in fetal heart rate with return to baseline. Onset, nadir, and recovery occur after the beginning, peak, and end of the contraction, respectively.

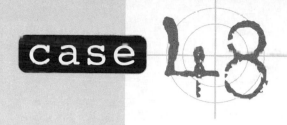

case 48

ID/CC A 17-year-old G1P0 at 37 weeks' gestation presents with severe **headache, blurry vision,** and dull right upper quadrant **abdominal pain** of 4 hours duration; while in the ambulance, she had a generalized tonic-clonic **seizure.**

HPI Otherwise healthy young Hispanic woman with poor prenatal care; dates are established by a sure last menstrual period (LMP). She last saw a physician 1 month ago when she went to an emergency room for hand and face **swelling.** At that time she was told to see an obstetrician because her blood pressure was high, but has been unable to do so because of difficult social issues.

PE VS: HR 102, **(BP 160/100);** afebrile. Funduscopy reveals AV nicking; lungs clear to auscultation; abdominal examination reveals a uterus with size smaller than dates; fetal tachycardia (HR 170); right upper quadrant tenderness; no hepatomegaly; leg edema 3+; brisk DTRs.

Labs CBC: Hct 41, Plts 256K. Cr 0.8, uric acid 6.4. ABGs: mild acidosis. UA: 3+ proteinuria. ALT 54, AST 60. PT, PTT, INR, and fibrinogen normal.

Imaging Biophysical profile reveals oligohydramnios. Fetal parts measure 4 weeks smaller than her presumed gestational age. CXR: normal, no evidence of aspiration pneumonia from her seizure. CT, head: cerebral edema; no focal lesion identified as cause for seizure.

OBSTETRICS

case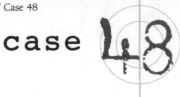

Eclampsia

Pathogenesis

Preeclampsia refers to a syndrome of **hypertension** (BP >140/90 on two occasions done 6 hours apart), and **proteinuria** (300 mg of protein in urine collected over a 24-hour period, ≥1+ protein or >30 mg/dL). **Edema** is no longer used as a diagnostic criterion. Preeclampsia develops after the 20th week of pregnancy. **Eclampsia** refers to **convulsions** in a preeclamptic woman that cannot be explained by any other etiology; 25% of eclampsia seizures occur antepartum, 50% intrapartum, and 25% postpartum. The etiology of preeclampsia is unknown, but women with existing hypertension, diabetes, or collagen vascular, autoimmune, or renal disease prior to pregnancy are at increased risk of developing preeclampsia and eclampsia.

Epidemiology

Occurs in approximately 1 in 2,000 pregnancies; more frequently seen among younger primigravidae of low socioeconomic groups and among Hispanics and blacks. Mortality is approximately 1%.

Management

For any seizure, begin ABCs (airway, breathing, and circulation). Prevent and treat convulsions with continuous intravenous **magnesium sulfate**. If diastolic BP >110 mm Hg, or systolic BP >170 to 180, hydralazine, nifedipine, or labetalol may be used to reduce stroke risk from the hypertensive emergency. The definitive treatment of eclampsia is **early delivery** through either induction of labor or cesarean section.

Complications

Fetal complications from eclampsia include placental abruption, premature delivery, and fetal or neonatal death. Maternal complications include airway obstruction, aspiration pneumonia, convulsions, fluid overload, hypoxia, hemorrhage, acute renal failure, hepatic capsule rupture, DIC, and maternal death.

Breakout Point

- Preeclampsia, eclampsia, and HELLP are different aspects of the same clinical entity. Thus, eclampsia and HELLP can be considered types of severe preeclampsia.
- Seizures after the 20th week of pregnancy should be presumed eclampsia unless imaging or labs indicate another cause.
- Expectant management of the very preterm patient with preeclampsia with close monitoring can be reasonable. However, if her condition worsens (increasing blood pressures, seizures, or end-organ damage), delivery is recommended.

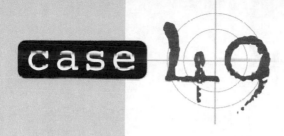

case 49

ID/CC A 32-year-old female presents with vaginal bleeding, **light-headedness,** nausea, vomiting, and **fainting** after **sudden-onset left lower quadrant abdominal pain** 2 hours ago; the pain radiates to the scapular region and to the back (diaphragmatic irritation due to tubal rupture).

HPI Several years ago, the patient was using an **IUD.** She has a history of **recurrent cervicitis and PID** due to *Neisseria gonorrhoeae* and had an appendectomy during childhood. Her **last menstrual period was 45 days ago,** but she states that she is regular and never misses a period.

PE VS: **tachycardia** (HR 110); **orthostatic hypotension (BP 100/60 seated, 80/40 standing);** tachypnea (RR 24); low-grade fever. PE: marked pallor; delayed capillary refill; abdomen distended; **tender left iliac fossa** with voluntary guarding and **rebound tenderness;** decreased bowel sounds; pelvic examination reveals mild **tenderness on cervical motion** and soft, **tender left adnexal mass;** culdocentesis reveals **nonclotting blood in cul-de-sac** (transvaginal ultrasound is replacing culdocentesis for diagnosis).

Labs CBC: mild anemia (due to intraperitoneal bleeding); leukocytosis. Lytes: normal. Increased BUN. UA: normal. Quantitative serial serum β-**hCG** shows prolonged doubling time, plateauing or decreasing levels (as compared with a normal pregnancy); blood type O negative.

Imaging Transvaginal ultrasound shows a **complex left adnexal mass.**

OBSTETRICS

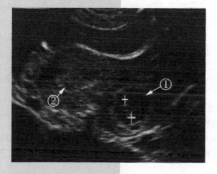

Figure 49-1. Transvaginal ultrasound showing the ectopic gestation sac (1) outside the empty uterus (2).

case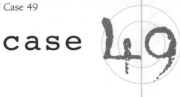

Ectopic Pregnancy

Pathogenesis

Ectopic pregnancy is **implantation of the fertilized ovum outside the uterine cavity,** usually in the ampullary region of the fallopian tubes, followed in frequency of occurrence by the isthmus, fimbria, and interstitial portion (part of the tube that traverses the uterine wall). Ova may also implant in the cervix, abdominal cavity, and ovaries. The classic triad in ectopic pregnancy consists of **lower abdominal pain, amenorrhea, and vaginal bleeding,** but this triad is not always found. Interstitial pregnancy ruptures later, with more profuse bleeding than other tubal pregnancies. Risk factors include **tubal ligation, PID** with scarring, **IUD** use, previous ectopic pregnancy, previous complicated appendicitis with peritonitis, endometriosis, multiparity, perimenopausal years, exposure to DES, and induction of ovulation.

Management

Transvaginal ultrasound should be done in any pregnant woman presenting with first-trimester bleeding or pelvic pain. For an unruptured ectopic pregnancy <3.5 cm, **methotrexate** may be given to induce abortion; an alternative is laparoscopic surgery, with removal of the product of conception by **salpingectomy.** Tubal rupture requires emergency laparotomy. If the mother is Rh negative, then administer RhoGAM to prevent Rh isoimmunization.

Breakout Point

- Most common site is at ampulla of oviduct (95%).
- Ultrasound showing intrauterine pregnancy effectively rules out ectopic pregnancy; it is rare to have both intrauterine and extrauterine gestation.
- Diagnosis is made with β-hCG >1,500, nonspecific adnexal mass (or gestational sac) seen on transvaginal ultrasound, and no intrauterine pregnancy.

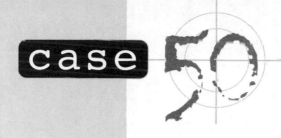

case 50

ID/CC	A 19-year-old G1P0 woman at **10 weeks** gestation by last menstrual period (LMP) presents to clinic with an **undesired pregnancy**.
HPI	She is in a relationship with the father of the baby, her boyfriend of 2 years, and they have discussed and agreed to proceed with **termination**. She has met with **social work** and understands all options available to her. She and her boyfriend had only been using condoms for birth control. She denies any significant past medical or surgical history. She **denies any vaginal bleeding, abdominal pain, or cramping**.
PE	VS: afebrile, stable. PE: speculum examination was performed. **Os was closed.** Gonorrhea and *Chlamydia* cultures were performed. Bimanual examination revealed a **9-week–sized nontender, anteverted uterus** with no adnexal masses noted.
Labs	Blood type = **A negative**, antibody negative, gonorrhea and *Chlamydia* negative.
Imaging	Transvaginal ultrasound confirmed an **intrauterine pregnancy with size equal to dates.**
Gross Pathology	**Immature placental villi** confirmed in pathology specimen.

■ TABLE 50-1 COMPLICATIONS OF ABORTION AND COMPLICATION RATES

Complications[a]	Surgical Regimens (%)[b]	Medical Regimens (%)[b]
Immediate postabortion		
Failure to dilate cervix	0.1	NA
Perforation	0.09–0.5	NA
Acute hematometra	0.1–1.0	NK
Anesthetic reaction, mild/severe	0.2	NA
Hemorrhage (>500 mL)	0.05–4.9	<1.0
Pain (moderate to severe)	0.5–5.0	10–30
Allergic reaction to medications	0.0–0.05	NK
Delayed		
Retained products of conception	0.5–1.0	4.0–7.0
Endometriosis/salpingitis/ infection	0.1–4.7	0.09–0.5
Transient fever	2.0	NK
Persistent positive β-hCG (>3 wks)	0.5–5.0	4.0–7.0
Continuing pregnancy	0.05	4.0–7.0[c]
Postabortion molar gestation	0.01–0.05	<1.0%
Long term		
Cervical injury	0.1–1.6	NA
Asherman syndrome, complete/partial	0.1–2.3	NK
Infertility	1.0–2.0	NK
Chronic pelvic inflammatory disease	1.0–2.0	NK
Psychological sequelae	0.5–1.0	NK

[a]Rates of serious complications <1/100.
[b]Estimates based on cumulative data in medical literature for a variety of gestational ages and procedures.
[c]Needs surgical abortion.
NA, not applicable; β-hCG, human chronic gonadotropins; NK, not yet known.

OBSTETRICS

case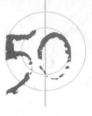

Elective Abortion

Pathogenesis Not applicable.

Management Antibiotic prophylaxis with **doxycycline** 100 mg PO 1 hour prior to procedure and 200 mg PO after the procedure. Given her gestational age, surgical management with **suction dilation and evacuation.** Medical management with regimens including **mifepristone, methotrexate, or misoprostol** would also have been options if she had been evaluated at an earlier gestational age. The upper limits of gestational age allowing for medical abortion range from **49 to 63 days**. No data exist to support universal use of prophylactic antibiotics for medical abortion. Also, because patient is **Rh negative**, it is crucial that she receive a **RhoGAM** shot (anti-D immune globulin) to prevent Rh isoimmunization in future pregnancies.

Complications Retained products of conception potentially requiring a second procedure, hemorrhage, infection, uterine perforation with possible damage to surrounding organs (bowel, bladder, blood vessels, nerves), psychosocial issues (e.g., regret or guilt).

Breakout Point

- Annually, approximately 2% of reproductive-aged women legally terminate a pregnancy in the United States.
- About one half of the 6 million pregnancies that occur each year in the United States are unplanned. Of those unplanned pregnancies, approximately half result in induced abortion.
- Abortion can be achieved using either medical and surgical techniques.

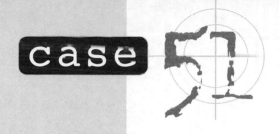
ID/CC	A 25-year-old G1P0 at **39 6/7** weeks gestation presents to Labor and Delivery with **regular painful contractions** of 4 hours duration, desiring pain management.
HPI	She also reports **leaking of clear fluid,** which began 1 hour ago, after which the **contractions became much stronger and more frequent.** She denies any vaginal bleeding. She reports active fetal movement.
PE	VS: Afebrile, BP 120/80, HR 98. PE: Patient **uncomfortable** and breathing through contractions. Abdomen is soft, nontender, and gravid. Sterile speculum examination reveals pooling of clear fluid in vaginal vault, nitrizine +, and ferning +. Sterile vaginal examination was **3 cm dilated, 100% effaced, −1 station.** Fetal heart tracing was reactive with baseline at 140s with moderate variability, + accelerations, no decelerations. Tocometer revealed **q2min contractions.**
Labs	O+, antibody negative, WBC 9.8, Hct 31.2, **platelets 220.**
Imaging	Not applicable.

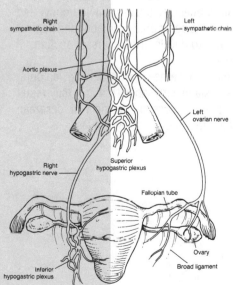

Figure 51-1. Sympathetic nerve supply of the uterus from the pelvic and abdominal distribution.

case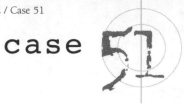

Epidural Anesthesia During Labor

Pathogenesis
Pain impulses are carried in visceral afferent type C fibers accompanying the sympathetic nerves. **Specific dermatomes are affected depending on the stage of labor.** Early labor only affects thoracic dermatomes **(T11-T12)** via the hypogastric plexus. With progressing cervical dilation, adjacent dermatomes also become involved **(T10-L1)**. Finally, with the second stage of labor, additional pain impulses secondary to distension of the vaginal vault and perineum are carried by the pudendal nerve **(S2-S4)**.

Management
IV placement followed by evaluation and epidural placement by the anesthesia team.

Complications
Hypotension, "high" spinal (level of anesthesia surpasses desired dermatome), inadvertent spinal anesthesia, ineffective anesthesia, **postdural puncture headache,** nerve injury, epidural abscess, epidural hematoma.

Breakout Point

- Epidural anesthesia can easily be converted from doses appropriate for labor and vaginal delivery to levels for cesarean section, if needed.
- Despite concerns that providing epidural anesthesia in early labor (<4 cm) may result in higher chances of dystocia or cesarean section, this has not been proven.

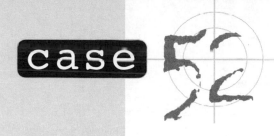

case 52

ID/CC A 35-year-old pregnant woman is admitted because of a **complicated obstetric history with gestational diabetes.**

HPI The patient is at 10 weeks' gestation. **During her first pregnancy she had gestational diabetes** and was prescribed insulin; her first pregnancy resulted in sudden unexpected fetal death at 36 weeks. Her second pregnancy resulted in a term **macrosomic infant weighing 4,500 g following a difficult vaginal delivery;** the baby suffered intraventricular hemorrhage and died shortly after birth. During both pregnancies, the patient had **irregular prenatal care and did not adhere to her insulin schedule. Her father is diabetic.**

PE VS: normal. PE: **obese;** pelvic examination reveals 10-week uterus; fetal heart heard on Doppler.

Labs Fasting blood **glucose 160 mg/dL** (if value is <140 mg/dL, retest at 24 to 28 weeks; if value is >140 mg/dL, proceed to glucose tolerance test). UA: **glucosuria. Glucose tolerance test results pending.**

Imaging US, pelvis: single, intrauterine fetus at 10 weeks with evidence of fetal heart activity.

■ TABLE 52-1 GLUCOSE SCREENING DURING PREGNANCY

Initial screening	50-g glucose load —> 1 hour glucose level	Negative: <140 (some physicians use 130 as cutoff)
If initial screen positive	3-hr oral glucose tolerance test	

case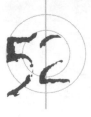

Gestational Diabetes

Pathogenesis

Gestational diabetes is caused by **insulin resistance during pregnancy** that is thought to be due to human placental lactogen (which blocks insulin receptors) and elevated circulating estrogen and progesterone. Risk factors include age (25 years or older), obesity, family history, symptoms of prior pregnancy consistent with gestational diabetes (infant >4,000 g, stillborn or congenitally deformed infant, polyhydramnios), and history of recurrent abortions.

Management

Gestational diabetes must be suspected in all women with a prior history of gestational diabetes; with **significant glucosuria** on two occasions prenatally or in a single fasting urine sample; with a family history of diabetes; with previous babies weighing >90th percentile for gestational age and sex; or with a history of previous unexpected perinatal death, polyhydramnios, or maternal obesity. **Routine prenatal screening is recommended at 24 to 28 weeks for all women and at initial visit for women with risk factors.** Prescribe the ADA diet; most cases of gestational diabetes may be managed with diet alone, but if needed, **insulin** may be used. **Oral hypoglycemics are contraindicated** during pregnancy because they cross the placenta and produce fetal hypoglycemia. Labor is generally induced at 38 to 40 weeks; with proper management, perinatal mortality can be decreased from 40% to about 5%. Women with gestational diabetes usually do not need insulin in the postpartum period, but are at increased risk of developing diabetes in the future; screen for diabetes 6 weeks postpartum.

Complications

Maternal risks include **retinopathy, nephropathy, neuropathy,** and increased risk of polyhydramnios, preeclampsia, and **UTIs.** **Fetal risks** include **congenital malformations** (cardiac and craniospinal defects); **sacral agenesis** (a rare anomaly specifically associated with diabetes); **sudden unexpected fetal death** during the last 4 to 6 weeks of pregnancy; difficult delivery (shoulder dystocia) due to **macrosomia;** and neonatal problems such as **birth trauma, hyaline membrane disease, hypoglycemia,** hypomagnesemia, **hypocalcemia,** and **jaundice.** All risks are increased by poor glycemic control, especially if ketoacidosis develops.

Breakout Point

- Strict glucose control leads to decreased maternal and fetal complications.
- C-section is used if expected fetal weight is >4,500 g.

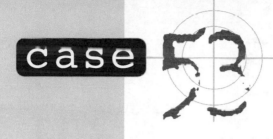

case 52

ID/CC A 38-year-old G1P0 at 38 weeks presents with **abdominal pain.**

HPI She woke up this morning with a mild pain in her right upper quadrant, which remained unchanged when she ate. Over the last 6 hours, the pain has worsened. She has had a normal antepartum course until now, although **her rings no longer fit** on her fingers. On review of systems, she notes a persistent **headache,** but no visual changes. She reports rare contractions, active fetal movement and denies loss of fluid or vaginal bleeding.

PE VS: BP 130/80. Abdominal examination reveals mild tenderness in the right upper quadrant, otherwise, her abdomen is soft with no rebound or guarding. The uterus measures size equaling dates. Neurologic examination demonstrates symmetrical hyperreflexia and no clonus. SVE is 1 cm dilated, long, and fix −3 station.

Labs Hct 38, **plts 96K,** ALT 65, AST 82, Cr 1.1, LDH 682; uric acid 8.4. UA: 1+ protein.

Imaging Biophysical profile reveals oligohydramnios. Peripheral blood smear shows **schistocytes.**

OBSTETRICS

case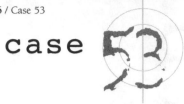

HELLP Syndrome

Pathogenesis	HELLP stands for **hemolysis, elevated liver enzymes, low platelets.** Preeclampsia develops after the twentieth week of pregnancy. The pathogenesis of HELLP syndrome is unclear, but it is felt to be a **part** of the **preeclampsia/eclampsia spectrum.** Preeclampsia refers to a syndrome of **hypertension** (BP . 140/90 on two occasions, 6 hours apart), and proteinuria (300 mg of protein in urine collected over a 24-hour period, >1+ protein or ≥30mg/dL). Edema is no longer used as a diagnostic criterion.
Management	Delivery, either by induction of labor or cesarean section. Because of increased risk for seizures, magnesium sulfate seizure prophylaxis should be started.
Complications	Eclampsia, cerebral hemorrhage, DIC, pulmonary edema, liver or renal failure, hepatic rupture, electrolyte abnormalities, coagulopathy, placental abruption, idiopathic premature delivery, maternal and fetal death.
Breakout Point	• HELLP stands for **h**emolysis, **e**levated **l**iver enzymes, **l**ow **p**latelets. • Preeclampsia, eclampsia, and HELLP are part of the same spectrum. • The only treatment for preeclampsia, eclampsia, and HELLP is stabilization of the mother and delivery of the fetus.

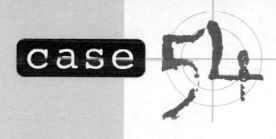

case 54

ID/CC	A 25-year-old woman, **HIV positive,** presents for her initial obstetric visit after a positive over-the-counter pregnancy test.
HPI	She was diagnosed with HIV 1 year ago, but did not start antiretroviral therapy. She has not experienced any opportunistic infections, and continues to work full time.
PE	VS normal. Well-appearing woman without abnormal lymphadenopathy.
Labs	CD4 800. HIV RNA viral count 1,500/mL.
Imaging	Not applicable.
Gross Pathology	Not applicable.
Micro Pathology	Not applicable.

OBSTETRICS

case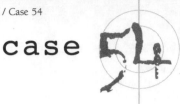

HIV Transmission in Pregnancy

Pathogenesis

With no treatment, **25% of infants** born of HIV-infected mothers will be infected with HIV. The risk is higher in higher viral burden (of mother), rupture of membranes, or other events during labor and delivery that increase the infant's exposure to maternal blood. Transmission takes place during labor/delivery or in late pregnancy.

Management

All expectant mothers should be offered HIV screening because transmission to the infant can be significantly decreased with appropriate management. Antiretrovi treatment for the mother should start/continue based on **CD4 and HIV RNA viral counts,** whether the patient is pregnant or not; but pregnant women may delay initiation of treatment until after 10 to 12 weeks of gestation. Combination antiretroviral therapy is recommended when the HIV RNA viral count is >1,000 copies/mL. **Cesarean delivery** (recommended at 38 weeks, and definitely prior to membrane rupture) and **zidovudine (AZT)** together reduce the transmission rate by about 85%. Prenatal procedures such as fetal blood sampling, invasive fetal monitoring, and artificial rupture of membranes should be minimized as they increase the risk of transmission. HIV-infected mothers should **avoid breastfeeding,** which could transmit the virus.

Breakout Point

- C-section and AZT reduce vertical transmission by 85%.
- Breastfeeding should be avoided.

■ TABLE 54-1 OPPORTUNISTIC INFECTION PROPHYLAXIS

CD4 Count	Prophylaxis
<200	*Pneumocystis carinii* pneumonia and toxoplasmosis (Bactrim)
<100	Mycobacterium avium complex (clarithromycin or azithromycin)

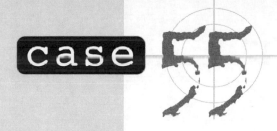

case 55

ID/CC   A 27-year-old **primigravida** complains of persistent, severe vomiting and **excessive morning nausea and vomiting** of 1 month's duration.

HPI   Five weeks ago she tested positive on a urine pregnancy test. She has been amenorrheic for 12 weeks, and her **food and water intake has been markedly reduced** owing to persistent nausea. She had a 7-pound weight loss over the past month.

PE   VS: Weight is down >5% from prepregnancy weight. **Tachycardia (HR 105); orthostatic hypotension.** PE: appears ill and moderately **dehydrated;** abdominal examination reveals fundal height to be at level of pelvic brim (12 weeks); fetal heart heard via Doppler.

Labs   Serum hCG elevated (commensurate with period of gestation). Lytes: **low Na, K, Cl.** Slightly elevated **free T4** with **low TSH** (up to 60% of women with severe hyperemesis gravidarum have a transient elevation of T4 due to thyroid-stimulating effect of hCG). **ALT and AST mildly elevated.** Normal bilirubin. Very mildly elevated amylase/lipase (from vomiting). UA: positive **ketones, elevated specific gravity.** Further blood tests confirm **ketonemia.**

Imaging   US, abdomen/pelvis: single, live intrauterine 12-week gestation with positive fetal heart activity. Normal liver and gallbladder.

■ **TABLE 55 1 DIFFERENTIAL DIAGNOSIS OF NAUSEA/VOMITING IN PREGNANCY**

Diagnosis	Key Distinguishing Clinical Diagnostic Features
Gastric mucosal irritation; NSAIDs, EtOH	Abd pain ↓ with eating
Appendicitis	Abd pain, tenderness, fever
Cholelithiasis/cholecystitis	Abd pain ↑ with eating, ↑ LFTs
Hepatitis	Abd pain, ↑ LFTs, icterus
Pancreatitis	Abd pain, ↑ lipase
Endocrine disorders: thyrotoxicosis, DKA, hyperparathyroidism or hypoparathyroidism, adrenal insufficiency	History, laboratory abnormalities

OBSTETRICS

case 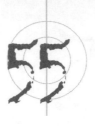 55

Hyperemesis Gravidarum

Pathogenesis

50%–90% of pregnant women experience some degree of nausea and/or vomiting. Symptoms usually **begin at 5 to 6 weeks, peak at 9 weeks, and abate by 16 to 18 weeks.** The cause of vomiting is thought to be high hCG levels. Elevated estrogen/progesterone levels, slowed gastric motility, and nutritional factors may be involved but are less well correlated. Hyperemesis gravidarum is defined by **severe nausea and vomiting leading to dehydration and electrolyte abnormalities.** There are no clear risk factors. Age >35 and smoking appear to be protective.

Management

Other causes of hyperemesis must be ruled out, including hyperthyroidism, GI disorders, multiple gestation, or molar pregnancy, as hyperemesis gravidarum is a diagnosis of exclusion. Mild symptoms may respond to ginger supplements, doxylamine (Unisom), and pyridoxine (vitamin B6). If necessary, **antiemetics** may be given. Administer **thiamine** to prevent Wernicke syndrome if patient has been vomiting for 3 or more weeks. Patients with severe cases may need feeding tubes or, as a last resort, parenteral nutrition. In very severe cases that are resistant to intensive therapy, termination of pregnancy may be required.

Complications

Electrolyte imbalance, nutritional deficiency, and their consequences, especially Wernicke encephalopathy from thiamine deficiency and bleeding from vitamin K deficiency. Overly rapid correction of hyponatremia may lead to central pontine myelinolysis. Mallory–Weiss tears, esophageal rupture, pneumothorax, and pneumomediastinum are less common. In advanced cases, **renal and hepatic function may be compromised** (known as the toxemic phase of vomiting).

Breakout Point

- Hyperemesis gravidarum is a diagnosis of exclusion, and includes weight loss, dehydration, electrolyte imbalance, and ketonuria.
- Hyperemesis gravidarum occurs in the first trimester and usually abates by mid–second trimester.

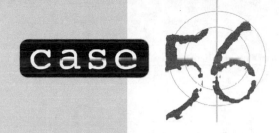

case 56

ID/CC	A 35-year-old G3P2 presents at 23 weeks' gestation (**second trimester**). She has a history of one-term NSVD, followed by fetal loss at 22 weeks, and then NSVD at 32 weeks. The patient was sent from clinic to Labor and Delivery after a transvaginal ultrasound done for vaginal spotting demonstrated an **endocervical canal length** of 12 mm (**<25 mm**) and **funneling of the cervix** (a sign that the cervix is beginning to efface).
HPI	The patient reports vaginal pressure but **no pain**. She also notes one day of **light vaginal spotting.** She denies abdominal pain, back pain, contractions, or vaginal discharge. She denies exposure to DES. She had a **cold knife cone biopsy** 3 years prior, after her first pregnancy.
PE	VS: normal. Sterile speculum examination shows no evidence of ruptured membranes. Fetal heart rate in the 130s; variability is appropriate for gestational age. Digital examination reveals a 1-cm dilated cervix, 80% effaced.
Labs	Wet mount is negative for bacterial vaginosis.
Imaging	Transvaginal ultrasound shows a shortened cervix (see HPI section) and no evidence of placenta previa.
Gross Pathology	Not applicable.
Micro Pathology	Not applicable.

OBSTETRICS

case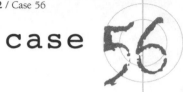

Incompetent Cervix

Pathogenesis

Cervical incompetence is a silent process and should be differentiated from preterm contractions or labor. The most common cause of cervical incompetence is **prior cervical surgery** (e.g., cone biopsy, LEEP, cervical dilatation) or **trauma** (including history of cervical laceration from vaginal delivery). Other causes include **uterine anomalies, DES exposure** in utero, deficiency in cervical collagen and elastin, and overdistension of the uterus as seen with multiple gestations or polyhydramnios. However, many presenting patients have no known risk factors, and history of cervical incompetence increases the risk of recurrence.

Management

Cervical **cerclage** (Fig. 56-1), wherein sutures are placed to reinforce the cervix, is the primary treatment for women presenting with previable pregnancies if there is adequate cervical length or the cervix is not too dilated (the degree of dilation depends on surgeon comfort). Cerclages are **removed at 36 to 38 weeks of gestation,** and then the patient is followed expectantly until labor starts. If vaginal cerclage fails, abdominal cerclage may be required. For women with a previous diagnosis of incompetent cervix, cerclage may be performed electively at 12 to 14 weeks of gestation. Other alternatives for the previable pregnancy include expectant management on bed rest or therapeutic abortion. When the incompetent cervix is diagnosed beyond 24 weeks of gestation (i.e., viable pregnancy), corticosteroids are administered (to decrease morbidity from preterm birth), and the patient is managed expectantly with bed rest.

Breakout Point

- Cervical incompetence is characterized by painless cervical dilatation.
- Most common causes are prior cervical surgery and trauma.

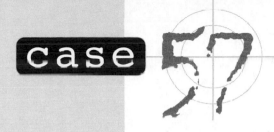

ID/CC A 31-year-old woman complains of **easy fatigability** and **lack of stamina for daily activities**; she has also had an unusual **urge to eat ice** (pagophagia) **and clay** (pica).

HPI She is a 20-week primigravida with an unremarkable medical history.

PE VS: mild tachycardia (HR 105). PE: **pallor** of mucous membranes; fetal heart rate normal (140/min).

Labs CBC: **microcytic, hypochromic** (MCHC <30) anemia (may be normochromic or normocytic with concomitant folate deficiency); low hematocrit. **Low serum iron level; low transferrin saturation index** (<16%); **increased TIBC; low ferritin level.** UA/Lytes: normal. Glucose normal.

Imaging US, abdomen: 20-week intrauterine pregnancy.

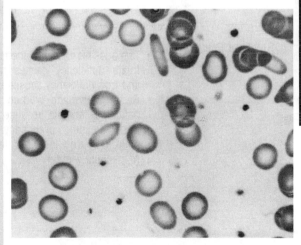

Figure 57-1. Peripheral blood smear showing hypochromic and microcytic RBCs with poikilocytosis.

OBSTETRICS

113

case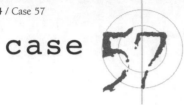

Iron Deficiency Anemia

Pathogenesis

Iron deficiency anemia is anemia (Hct <30% or Hb <10 g/dL) caused by lack of iron, resulting from diminished consumption, decreased absorption, increased demand (short interval between pregnancies), blood loss (hemorrhage), or a combination thereof. In pregnancy, iron absorption is usually increased (as opposed to folate) to offset increased demand. Because ferritin is the storage form of iron, **ferritin level is the test of choice in the diagnosis of iron deficiency** anemia.

Management

All pregnant women should take low-dose iron supplementation; this is contained in prenatal vitamin preparations and suffices for prophylaxis of overt anemia. If iron deficiency anemia is established, 325 mg of ferrous sulfate should be given three times a day. Administration of iron together with vitamin C increases absorption; taking it with antacids, calcium, or meals decreases absorption. Iron-dextran may be given IM if a patient cannot tolerate iron PO.

Breakout Point

- Two possible causes of anemia during pregnancy: folate deficiency causes macrocytic anemia, and iron deficiency causes microcytic anemia.
- Reproductive-age women may develop iron deficiency anemia because of excessive menstrual bleeding, pregnancy, lactation (another source of iron loss), or lack of dietary iron (especially vegetarians).

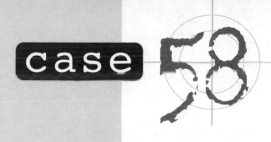

case 58

ID/CC	A 30-year-old G1P0 at **8 3/7 weeks** gestation by LMP confirmed by first-trimester ultrasound, presents for her initial prenatal visit.
HPI	She is feeling well overall except for significant **fatigue**. She reports occasional episodes of **light-headedness** and has noticed **decreased exercise tolerance**. She also reports nausea, especially in the mornings, with only occasional episodes of emesis.
PE	VS: stable. PE: mild **pallor** of skin; otherwise, examination normal.
Labs	Hemoglobin 8.5 g/dL, MCV 100, folate 2.5 ng/mL. Peripheral blood smear notable for **hypersegmented neutrophils**.

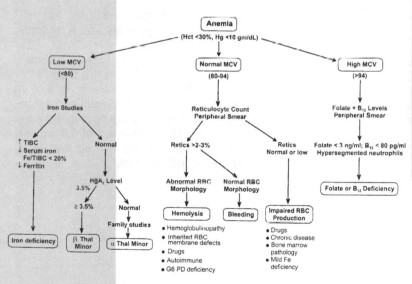

Figure 58-1. Workup of anemia in pregnancy.

OBSTETRICS

case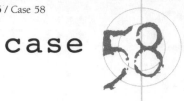

Megaloblastic Anemia of Pregnancy (Folate Deficiency)

Pathogenesis

Folate deficiency can develop over a fairly short period of time because the liver's folate stores can only meet the body's needs for **1 to 2 months.** Pregnancy, malnutrition (e.g., alcoholism), malabsorption, anticonvulsant therapy, and oral contraceptive use can rapidly deplete the folate stores.

Management

Folic acid supplementation—0.5 to 1 mg/day is recommended for treatment of deficiency.

Complications

Potential for **neural tube defects** in infants if deficiency is notable at beginning of pregnancy during early fetal development.

Breakout Point

- Megaloblastic anemia complicates approximately 1% of pregnancies and is typically caused by folate deficiency.
- Daily folate requirement for a pregnant woman is 0.4 mg (which is >4 times that required for nonpregnant women).
- Folic acid is important to prevent neural tube defects. Women contemplating pregnancy are advised to take a supplement of 0.4 mg/day prior to pregnancy and continued at least through the first trimester.

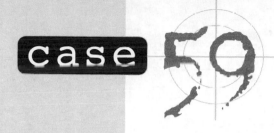

case 59

ID/CC	A 67-year-old G4P4 complains of a **heavy sensation** in her lower abdomen that becomes more pronounced toward the end of the day and if she strains. She also notes increased frequency of urination and dysuria.
HPI	She is an otherwise healthy **multiparous** female whose children were delivered vaginally. She has been **menopausal** for 15 years and has not taken hormone replacement.
PE	Inspection of external genitalia reveals a **cervix protruding 1 cm beyond the hymenal ring.** During Valsalva maneuver, the cervix protrudes further and the anterior wall of the vagina descends into the canal. She also leaks urine during Valsalva. The vaginal mucosa is keratinized.
Labs	UA: notable for leukoesterase and nitrates. UCx grows *E. Coli*
Imaging	Not applicable.
Gross Pathology	Not applicable.
Micro Pathology	Not applicable.

OBSTETRICS

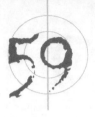

case 59

Pelvic Organ Prolapse

Pathogenesis

Pelvic floor prolapse is a **hernia of one of the pelvic organs (uterus, vaginal apex, bladder, rectum)** and its associated vaginal segment from its normal location. Risk factors include multiparity, operative vaginal delivery, obesity, advanced age, estrogen deficiency, neurogenic dysfunction of the pelvic floor, connective tissue disorders, prior pelvic surgery with disruption of natural support, and chronically increased intra-abdominal pressure from coughing or vigorous exercise.

Epidemiology

Most common in **multiparous, postmenopausal women.**

Management

Nonsurgical treatment includes avoidance of straining and lifting heavy weights, pessary support, local estrogen therapy, and pelvic floor exercises (**Kegel exercises**). Mild and moderate prolapse can be treated in this manner. Surgery, such as hysterectomy and colporrhaphy, is indicated for severe prolapse or if the patient fails nonsurgical interventions.

Complications

Keratinization and ulceration of the vagina and cervix, difficulties with urination and defecation, recurrent urinary tract infections.

Breakout Point

- Pelvic organ prolapse occurs with the relaxation of the pelvic floor, involving the pelvic floor musculature, fascial supports, and nervous system.
- Pelvic organ prolapse is not a life-threatening disease, but a quality-of-life issue.
- Mild prolapse can be treated with Kegel exercises and physical therapy; moderate prolapse and nonsurgical candidates may benefit from pessary placement; surgery is recommended for severe prolapse.

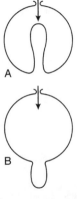

Figure 59-1. A. Intraabdominal pressure (arrow) on the uterus results in B. Uterine prolapse with the cervix extending 3 cm below the hymen.

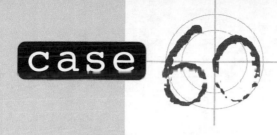
case 60

ID/CC A 30-year-old primigravida is brought to the emergency room with **continuous, painful vaginal bleeding.**

HPI On admission, she began to **bleed from her IV site and from her nose.** She is calculated to be at 35 weeks' gestation and admits to **smoking** and **abusing cocaine;** she has also been hypertensive (cocaine induced) for the past month. She has had no prior episodes of similar vaginal bleeding but has a history of **physical abuse** by her husband.

PE VS: **hypotension** (BP 90/50); **tachycardia** (HR 115). PE: looks extremely ill; epistaxis noted; abdominal examination reveals **tense uterus with marked tenderness; fetal heart audible but bradycardic** (HR 95); heavily blood-stained sanitary pad in place. Frequent contractions noted on tocometer.

Labs CBC/PBS: **thrombocytopenia;** fragmented RBCs. Coagulation profile reveals **prolonged clot retraction time, elevated fibrinogen degradation products, hypofibrinogenemia, prolonged PT/PTT and thrombin time,** and decreased antithrombin III and plasminogen.

Imaging Abdominal ultrasound: significant **placental abruption with a large retroplacental clot.** No previa noted. FHR confirmed in the 90s.

Gross Pathology At time of cesarean section, the entire uterus appears matted and purplish (Couvelaire uterus). There is a large 7-cm retroplacental clot noted.

Micro Pathology Villi are notably separated from the underlying deciduas basalis, and there exists an intramyometrial infiltration of blood and clot formation.

OBSTETRICS

119

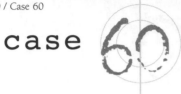

case

Placental Abruption

Pathogenesis

Placental abruption is caused by **premature separation of a normally implanted placenta before the third stage of labor.**

Epidemiology

The incidence of placental abruption is 1%; it is classified into marginal, partial, or total abruption and is the second most common cause of third-trimester bleeding. **Predisposing factors** include **preeclampsia, history of previous abruption, chronic hypertension, advanced maternal age, smoking and cocaine abuse, abdominal trauma, and sudden decrease in uterine volume** (such as that caused by ruptured membranes in polyhydramnios or after delivery of the first twin).

Management

Hydrate and correct bleeding complications with, packed red blood cells, fresh frozen plasma, and cryoprecipitate (for replacement of fibrinogen if bleeding complications occur) replacement. Immediate delivery by cesarean section in cases of severe bleeding or fetal distress, as in this patient. Address coagulation defects to limit bleeding during the delivery and in the postpartum period.

Complications

Hemorrhagic shock (sometimes due to concealed hemorrhage into a large retroplacental clot), coagulopathy (DIC occurs in 3% of severe abruptions), ischemic necrosis of distant organs (ATN, Sheehan syndrome), postpartum hemorrhage, increased risk of recurrence in subsequent pregnancies, fetal anemia, and fetal death.

Breakout Point

- Painful third-trimester vaginal bleeding is noted in 80% of patients with placental abruption.
- Diagnosis is made on a clinical basis. Ultrasound may detect large abruptions, however it is not sensitive enough to outweigh clinical suspicion.

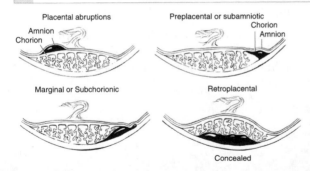

Placental abruptions
Amnion
Chorion

Preplacental or subamniotic
Chorion
Amnion

Marginal or Subchorionic

Retroplacental

Concealed

Figure 60-1. Diagrammatic representation of various degrees of placental abruption. Preplacental or subamnionic (between the amnion and chorion), marginal or subchorionic (between placenta and membranes), retroplacental (between placenta and myometrium), and concealed.

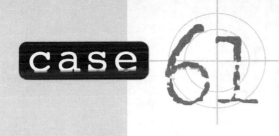

case 67

ID/CC	A 28-year-old multipara at **34 weeks and 2 days** gestation presents with **painless, moderate vaginal bleeding**.
HPI	Patient reports that bleeding began several hours ago and that she has felt **no contractions or loss of amniotic fluid**. She has had recurrent episodes of small amounts of vaginal bleeding, with first episode at about 28 weeks (**sentinel bleed**). These episodes are not preceded by trauma or intercourse, and resolve spontaneously. She was told that her fetal survey at 16 weeks revealed a low-lying placenta.
PE	VS: normal. PE: uterus relaxed with no contractions. **Vaginal examination not performed** to prevent provocation of further bleeding or hemorrhage. **Gentle speculum examination** show a moderate amount of bright red blood in the vagina.
Labs	**CBC and coagulation panel:** normal. **Rh typing** for possible use of Rhogam. Blood grouping sent and cross-matched in preparation for possible need of transfusion.
Imaging	Transabdominal **ultrasound** shows a viable fetus with **low anterior placenta**. Gentle transvaginal ultrasound shows the edge of the placenta overlaps the cervical internal os. Biophysical profile suggests fetal well-being. Review of the 20-week fetal survey reveals a partial placenta previa as well.
Gross Pathology	Not applicable.
Micro Pathology	Not applicable.

case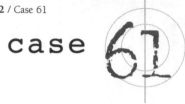

Placenta Previa

Pathogenesis

Placenta previa is defined as the **abnormal implantation of the placenta to cover the cervical os.** There are three types: **total** (internal os entirely covered), **partial** (as in this case), and **marginal** (edge of placenta reaches the os). Hemorrhage is caused by **disruption of placental vessels** as the internal os dilates and is enhanced by the inability of the lower uterine segment to contract. This can occur anytime within the second half of pregnancy, but often occurs after 28 weeks.

Epidemiology

Placenta previa occurs in **approximately 1 in 300** deliveries, increasing in patients with **advanced maternal age, prior cesarean delivery, smoking, multiparity,** and **multigestational** pregnancies.

Management

Management of placenta previa depends largely on the **extent of bleeding and fetal maturity.** If bleeding has stopped and fetus is not yet viable, then careful observation and pelvic rest may be all that is required. **Betamethasone** can be given to promote fetal lung maturity if patient is between 24 and 34 weeks of gestation to prepare for possible emergent delivery. If bleeding is stopped but the fetus is of appropriate maturity, then **elective cesarean delivery** should be considered to reduce risk to both mother and fetus. If bleeding is severe or fetus is unstable, then **emergent cesarean delivery** is required.

Complications

Bleeding can be severe and lead to hemorrhagic shock, and maternal/fetal demise. Preterm delivery (neonatal mortality increased 3-fold). Fetal growth restriction.

Breakout Point

- Placenta previa is abnormal placental implantation covering the cervical os.
- The bleeding caused by placenta previa is maternal. Patients with unstable placenta previa should have blood ready for possible transfusion.

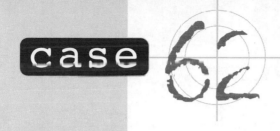

case 62

ID/CC	A 28-year-old G2P1001 woman presents to a family clinic with **weight gain** and **difficulty breathing**.
HPI	Her **last menstrual period was 24 weeks ago.** She had a normal full-term pregnancy and delivered a healthy male baby vaginally 3 years ago; she has no history of any abortions or stillbirths. She has no history of diabetes or hypertension, and her blood group is B positive. Her current pregnancy was diagnosed at home via urine testing, and she sought **no prenatal care.** She has not been taking prenatal vitamins.
PE	VS: tachycardia (HR 105); normal BP; tachypnea (RR 24). PE: no pallor, icterus, or pedal edema; abdominal examination reveals markedly distended abdomen; **fundal height corresponds to 32 weeks'** gestation (calculated at 24 weeks); **fluid thrill** palpable in all directions; **distant fetal heart sounds** audible.
Labs	Serum **α-fetoprotein (AFP)** (ideally should have been done at 15 to 20 weeks of gestation) **elevated; screening test for gestational diabetes negative.**
Imaging	Abdominal ultrasound: **amniotic fluid index greater than 25** and **anencephalic fetus.**
Gross Pathology	Anencephaly confirmed at autopsy after delivery.

OBSTETRICS

case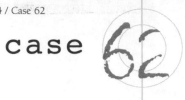

Polyhydramnios

Pathogenesis

Polyhydramnios means excessive amniotic fluid, associated with fetal polyuria or decreased swallowing by the fetus. Although its exact cause is not known, it is strongly associated with the following: **maternal diabetes twin–twin transfusion syndrome** (in which the hydramnios affects only one amniotic sac); **neural tube defects** such as anencephaly and spina bifida; hydrops fetalis related to Rh isoimmunization. **Polyhydramnios is present in half of cases in which there there is an open defect allowing free communication with the CSF.**

Epidemiology

Polyhydramnios affects 1% of all pregnancies.

Management

Perform frequent US examinations. Consider therapeutic amniocentesis in the presence of maternal respiratory compromise/marked uterine distention. Tocolysis if premature labor ensues; deliver if fetus is mature. To detect neural tube defects, **maternal serum AFP is recommended as a routine screening prenatal test at 15 to 18 weeks of pregnancy. Folic acid supplementation** (4 mg/day) is recommended for the next pregnancy to reduce the risk of neural tube defects.

Complications

Preterm labor, maternal respiratory distress, PPROM, umbilical cord prolapse, abruptio placentae, and fetal malpresentation.

Breakout Point

- Polyhydramnios means excessive amniotic fluid.
- 20% of polyhydramnios cases are related to maternal diabetes mellitus.

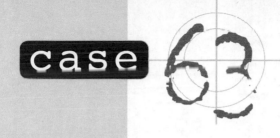

case 63

ID/CC A 43-year-old G5P5 presents with **excessive bleeding following spontaneous vaginal delivery** of a healthy baby girl.

HPI The placenta is delivered spontaneously 25 minutes after delivery. Thirty minutes after delivery, the patient continues to bleed heavily with a total estimated blood loss of 900 mL. She is hypotensive and requires fluid resuscitation. Preparations are made for blood transfusion.

PE VS: no fever; hypotension (BP 85/50); tachycardia (HR 120). Palpation of uterus reveals **soft, enlarged, boggy uterus.** Inspection of the cervix and vagina reveals no visible lacerations.

Labs CBC: anemia (Hgb 10.2); platelets normal. PT/PTT/INR normal.

Imaging Not applicable.

case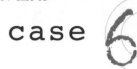

Postpartum Hemorrhage

Pathogenesis

Postpartum hemorrhage is defined as blood loss >500 mL after vaginal delivery and >1,000 mL after cesarean section. Common causes of postpartum hemorrhage include the **"4 Ts": tone, tissue, trauma, and thrombosis. Tone** refers to **uterine atony** (the most common cause of postpartum hemorrhage). Failure of the myometrial muscles to contract can lead to rapid and severe hemorrhage. **Tissue** refers to retained products of conception (RPOC). Careful inspection of the placenta should always be performed to ensure complete separation, as complete detachment and expulsion is needed for uterine contraction and optimal occlusion of the blood vessels. **Trauma** refers to damage of the genital tract during delivery of the baby, including uterine rupture, uterine inversion, cervical and vaginal lacerations, and hematomas. Finally, **thrombosis** refers to coagulation disorders and platelet abnormalities.

Management

Initial management of postpartum hemorrhage requires aggressive restoration of circulating blood volume with fluid resuscitation and blood transfusion. Uterine atony is treated with **oxytocin** infusion and **bimanual massage of the uterus** to assist the uterus in contraction. Underlying coagulopathies should be corrected with fresh frozen plasma, cryoprecipitate, and platelets. **D&C** may be necessary for treatment of refractory bleeding. In some cases, **laparotomy** (to ligate the uterine blood supply, or to adequately contract the uterus) and hysterectomy may be needed. If the patient is hemodynamically stable but still continues to bleed, **uterine artery embolization** may be an option to avoid hysterectomy.

Complications

Severe postpartum hemorrhage may result in massive blood loss and hypovolemic shock with organ failure. Sheehan syndrome (anterior pituitary infarction) may also occur.

Breakout Point

- Postpartum hemorrhage: blood loss >500 mL after vaginal delivery or > 1,000 mL after cescreail section.
- Common causes are the 4 T's: tone, tissue, trauma, thrombosis.

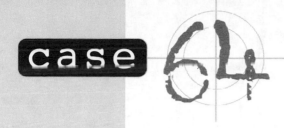

case 64

ID/CC A 30-year-old G1P1001 woman presents with **fever, malaise**, and **lower abdominal pain** 5 days **following a cesarean section**.

HPI Her **lochia (uterine discharge) has become purulent** and is particularly **foul-smelling**. She denies any breast discomfort, dysuria, cough, or any painful injection sites; the baby is healthy.

PE VS: tachycardia (HR 110); mild tachypnea (RR 20); normal BP; **fever (38.9°C)**. PE: breast examination normal, chest examination normal; **uterine tenderness**; lochia staining pad is purulent and foul smelling; surgical wound clean, dry, and intact.

Labs CBC: **leukocytosis**. UA: trace albumin. **High vaginal swab was stained and cultured**; Gram stain reveals gram-positive cocci and gram-negative bacilli; culture shows **group B streptococci, E. coli, and anaerobic peptostreptococci**; blood culture is sterile.

Imaging Pelvic US: no evidence of retained products of conception, normal postoperative changes are noted.

Gross Pathology Not applicable.

Micro Pathology Not applicable.

OBSTETRICS

case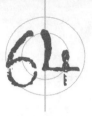

Postpartum Infection

Pathogenesis

Postpartum infection is often caused by normal bacteria in the vaginal flora or from exogenous pathogens. Normal vaginal flora may become pathogenic during the puerperium because of alteration in normal defenses. Diagnosis is clinical with findings of fever (>100.4°F, or 38°C, for at least 2 of the first 10 days of the puerperium, excluding the first 24 hours), elevated WBC count, and uterine tenderness.

Epidemiology

Risk factors include **early rupture of the membranes, prolonged labor, numerous vaginal examinations, use of internal monitoring devices, and instrumental and operative deliveries such as cesarean section.**

Management

Antibiotic treatment typically includes a combination of broad-spectrum antibiotics to provide coverage against gram-negative bacilli, gram-positive cocci, and anaerobes. Gentamicin and clindamycin are considered standard therapy. Occasionally penicillins or cephalosporins are also added to provide further coverage. Heparin is administered for septic pelvic thrombophlebitis (which is a diagnosis of exclusion). In addition to antibiotics, **D&C may be required** to remove retained products of conception, if present.

Complications

Sepsis, acute renal failure, septic pelvic thrombophlebitis, shock, and death.

Breakout Point

- The most common cause of postpartum fever is uterine infection, endomyometritis, which affects 1% to 3% of patients following vaginal delivery and up to 27% of patients following cesarean section.
- Diagnostic criteria for endomyometritis include elevated white blood cell count, foul-smelling or purulent lochia, fever, fundal tenderness, and absence of any other obvious infection.
- Typically, initial signs of postpartum infection will be evident within the first 5 days after delivery.

■ TABLE 64-1 MAJOR RISK FACTORS FOR POSTPARTUM INFECTION

Duration of labor
Cesarean delivery, especially nonelective
Nonelective cesarean delivery, without prophylactic antibiotics
Duration of rupture of membranes
Failure to progress in labor
Number of vaginal examinations
Duration of internal fetal monitoring
Low socioeconomic status
Diabetes

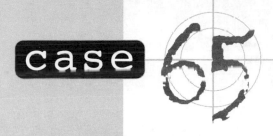

case 65

ID/CC	An **18-year-old pregnant** woman presents to the clinic after a positive home pregnancy test. Her last menstrual period was approximately 12 weeks ago.
HPI	She denies any previous sexually transmitted disease and is otherwise healthy. This is her first pregnancy and she is understandably anxious.
PE	VS: normal. PE: abdomen nontender, nondistended. Pelvic examination: no vaginal bleeding or discharge, no vaginal masses, **cervical os closed.**
Labs	See Table 65-1.

■ **TABLE 65-1 ROUTINE PRENATAL VISITS AND SCREENING (every 4 weeks for the first 28 weeks, every 2 weeks until 36 weeks, and weekly thereafter)**

First visit (usually between 6 and 10 weeks) Wt, BP, fundal height, fetal HR, and urinalysis for glucose and protein are obtained at every visit Average prenatal visits = 12	**History:** LMP, previous pregnancies, abortions and complications, STDs, HIV, varicella, social and family history **Physical:** height, weight, BP, uterine size and fundal height, cervical examination, bony pelvis for adequacy **Labs:** urine or serum β-hCG, urinalysis and urine culture, CBC with diff, RPR, rubella, HBsAg, HIV screening (if indicated), blood type, Rh type, cervical cultures for gonorrhea and *Chlamydia,* Pap smear **Counseling:** diet, medications, alcohol, smoking, drugs, x-rays, radiation, prenatal vitamins and folate
Weeks 6–12 (second visit)	Measure uterine size and growth via pelvic, fetal heart Doppler (after 10 weeks), chorionic villus sampling (if indicated)
Weeks 12–18	Amniocentesis (if indicated)
Weeks 18–22	Fetal ultrasound for dating and anatomy (biparietal diameter (BPD), head circ, abdominal circ, femur length). Earlier ultrasound = most accurate dating
Weeks 16–20	Serum AFP, estriol, and hCG (triple screen) to screen for neural tube defects and Down syndrome
Weeks 20–24	Educate about preterm labor and rupture of membranes.
Weeks 24–28	Repeat ultrasound (if needed)
Weeks 26–28	Gestational diabetes screen (Glucola; if positive, follow with 3-hr glucose tolerance test), and repeat Rh typing, if negative
Weeks 28 until labor and delivery	Repeat CBC for anemia and determine fetal position and presentation
Weeks 36 until labor and delivery	Repeat syphilis, HIV, gonorrhea, and *Chlamydia* testing in high-risk pts. Group B strep swab (abx with labor, if positive.) Discuss hospital plans, admission, labor, anesthesia, elective delivery
Beyond 41 weeks	Examine cervix, and discuss induction of labor, as needed

OBSTETRICS

129

case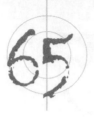

Prenatal Care

Pathogenesis | Not applicable.

Management | During the first prenatal visit, the physician should familiarize the patient with the process of pregnancy, especially those pregnant for the first time. Necessary prenatal testing should be discussed, as well as possible symptoms at each trimester. Pregnancy needs to be confirmed with β-hCG. Patients with significant nausea or vomiting and poor caloric intake should be referred to a nutritionist. A schedule of routine prenatal visits and testing is summarized in Table 65-1.

Breakout Point

> • "Gestational age" is dated from last menstrual period. "Developmental age" is dated from fertilization, and so is 2 weeks behind gestational age.
> • Ultrasound dating of pregnancy, if done in the first trimester, should come within 1 week of dating by last menstrual period.

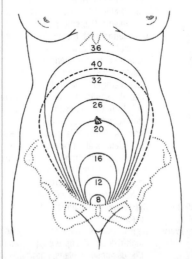

Figure 65-1. Fundal height during gestation. At 20 weeks the fundus is approximately at the umbilicus.

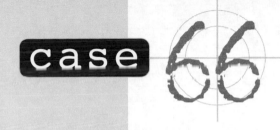

case 66

ID/CC	A 33-year-old G1 at 33 weeks and 1 day gestation presents with 3 hours of low **abdominal cramping** pain and passing **blood-tinged mucous.**
HPI	She has received routine prenatal care, and has had no complications this pregnancy. Denies vaginal bleeding or loss of fluid, and reports good fetal movement. She is having contractions every 3 minutes.
PE	VS: normal. Abdomen is soft and nontender. Her uterus in between contractions is also nontender. Sterile speculum examination shows no pool of fluid. The cervix is visibly dilated, and mucous is noted at cervical os. After a fetal fibronectin swab is collected, sterile vaginal examination shows cervix is 2 cm/ 100%/−2 station. Fetal heart tracing is reassuring.
Labs	Group B streptococcal culture is negative. Fetal fibronectin is positive.
Imaging	Abdominal ultrasound shows a viable fetus of approximately 33 weeks' gestation.
Gross Pathology	Not applicable.
Micro Pathology	Not applicable.

OBSTETRICS

case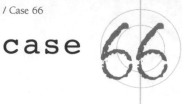

Preterm Labor

Pathogenesis

Preterm labor is defined as **labor before 37 weeks of gestation.** The exact cause of labor onset is unknown. However, risk factors for preterm labor include previous preterm delivery, uterine overdistension, multiple gestations, uterine anomalies, preterm rupture of membranes, chorioamnionitis or other infections, placental abruption, preeclampsia, and maternal prepregnancy weight of less than 50 kg.

Management

For patients with preterm contractions but no cervical change, **hydration** (by decreasing the level of ADH, which cross-reacts with oxytocin receptors to cause contractions) may decrease the number and strength of contractions. **Corticosteroids** (e.g., **betamethasone**) are given when preterm labor occurs before 34 weeks of gestation to reduce the incidence of infant respiratory distress syndrome, necrotizing enterocolitis, and intraventricular hemorrhage in the event of preterm delivery. **Tocolytics,** which halt contractions and the progression of labor, are used primarily to delay delivery by 48 hours, to allow the corticosteroids to take effect. In cases of chorioamnionitis, nonreassuring fetal testing, or preeclampsia, tocolysis is not appropriate and immediate delivery is required. For future pregnancies, prophylactic progesterone may be recommended to help prevent future preterm labor and delivery.

Complications

Preterm birth may result, which is the leading cause of neonatal mortality and morbidity in the United States. Prematurity increases the risk of infant respiratory distress syndrome, intraventricular hemorrhage, sepsis, and necrotizing enterocolitis.

Breakout Point

- Preterm delivery is delivery before 37 weeks gestation.
- Preterm delivery occurs in >10% of all pregnancies.
- Infants born at the cusp of viability (around 24 weeks of gestation) have a mortality rate of 50% or more. Infants born after 36 weeks have a mortality rate similar to that of full-term infants.
- Contractions alone are insufficient for the diagnosis of preterm labor; there must also be cervical change.

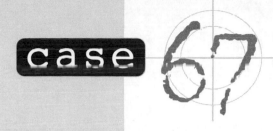

case 67

ID/CC	A 30-year-old at 30-weeks gestation presents to the emergency room with acute-onset **shortness of breath** with **left-sided pleuritic chest pain.**
HPI	First pregnancy in otherwise healthy woman. Because of a complicated prenatal course thus far, the patient has been on bed rest for 2 weeks.
PE	T 99.0°F, HR 105, Shallow breathing due to pleuritic pain. Lungs are clear to auscultation. **Bilateral lower extremity swelling** without a palpable cord.
Labs	CBC/Lytes normal. D-dimer is elevated.
Imaging	Doppler ultrasound shows no DVT. CT results pending.

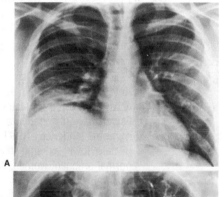

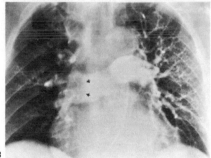

Figure 67-1. (A) Plain chest radiograph demonstrates right basilar atelectasis associated with elevation of the right hemidiaphragm, representing a large subpulmonic pleural effusion. **(B)** Pulmonary arteriogram shows virtually complete obstruction of the right pulmonary artery (*arrows*)

case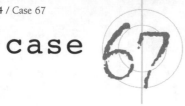

Pulmonary Embolus in Pregnancy

Pathogenesis

The Virchow triangle (risk factors for thromboembolic disease) is hypercoagulable state (pregnancy, cancer), stasis, and endothelial injury. Delivery is associated with vascular injury; therefore, thromboembolic disease is more common postpartum than antepartum.

Management

Warfarin is teratogenic when used between the sixth and ninth weeks of gestation, and also increases the risk of fetal hemorrhage during delivery. Unfractionated **heparin** or low-molecular-weight heparin (LMW heparin) are safe to use during pregnancy. It is also acceptable to start with unfractionated heparin or LMW heparin, switch to warfarin from the thirteenth week until the middle of the third trimester, and then switch back until delivery. If unfractionated heparin is used, PTT should be checked weekly.

Breakout Point

- Antepartum DVT/PE is equally distributed across the three trimesters.
- Fewer than 30% patients with PE have radiographic evidence of DVT at presentation.
- Bilateral lower extremity edema is common in normal pregnant women, and does not signify bilateral DVT.

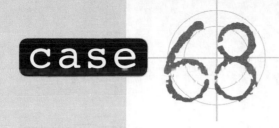

case 68

ID/CC   A **36-year-old** pregnant woman has an uncle with Down syndrome. She asks if she should be screened for genetic conditions.

HPI   Patient is otherwise healthy and her **spouse** has **no history of heritable diseases** in his family.

PE   VS: normal. Anxious woman. No other notable physical exam finding.

Labs   Alpha-fetoprotein (**AFP**), β-hCG, **unconjugated estriol** measurements, **inhibin-A.**

Imaging   Not applicable.

case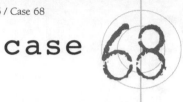

Quadruple Screen

Pathogenesis

Most cases of neural tube defects (NTDs), Down syndrome (trisomy 21), and other genetic abnormalities happen in **families with no history** of such conditions, so **all pregnant women** should be offered quadruple screening. **Maternal age** is factored in with a likelihood ratio calculated using all screening lab values to determine the possibility of an abnormality. Alpha-fetoprotein (**AFP**), β-hCG, **unconjugated estriol** measurements constitute the "triple screen," which is usually offered in the **second trimester**. **Inhibin-A** increases the sensitivity in the detection of Down syndrome, and was recently added to make the **quadruple screen;** this noninvasive panel of tests detects >80% of Down syndrome pregnancies. Any woman with increased risk (**age >35, abnormal US, previous fetal trisomy or chromosomal anomaly, parental chromosomal anomalies**) should be counseled for fetal karyotyping. Race, body weight, diabetes mellitus, multiple gestation, in vitro fertilization, and previous false-positive results are also factored into the calculations.

Management

Low AFP, elevated hCG, decreased serum estriol, and elevated inhibin-A suggest **Down syndrome.** Ultrasound should be used to confirm fetal age. Amniocentesis should be offered for karyotyping. **Parental counseling** after positive diagnosis is crucial. Elevated AFP indicates possible neural tube defect. Encephalic abnormalities are generally lethal, whereas isolated spinal defects may warrant pediatric neurology and neurosurgery consultation possible correction or counseling.

Breakout Point

- Down syndrome: low AFP, high β-hCG, low estriol, and high inhibin-A.
- Neural tube defect: high AFP.

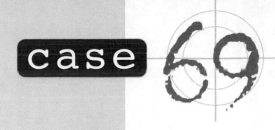

case 69

ID/CC A 35-year-old woman complains of **infrequent menstrual cycles** occurring at >42-day intervals (OLIGOMENORRHEA), coupled with **cold intolerance, coarse hair,** episodes of sweating with light-headedness and weakness (due to hypoglycemia), **weight loss** (6 kg in 3 months), and a feeling of constant **fatigue.**

HPI The patient suffered an **abruptio placentae** 7 years ago (average delay for onset of symptoms), with **severe bleeding** followed by **hypovolemic shock.** She had **failure of lactation** and quick breast involution (most common presenting sign) following the pregnancy. She had **persistent amenorrhea** for a year.

PE VS: **hypotension** (BP 100/50); tachycardia (HR 104); no fever. PE: dry skin; **coarse hair;** slow speech; thick tongue; periorbital swelling; **delayed relaxation phase of DTRs,** especially ankle (due to hypothyroidism); **lack of axillary and pubic hair** (due to adrenal insufficiency); vaginal examination reveals atrophic mucosa (due to lack of gonadotropin).

Labs CBC: normocytic, normochromic anemia; lymphocytosis; eosinophilia (due to adrenal insufficiency). **Low prolactin and cortisol; low T$_4$ and estradiol levels; low ACTH and TSH; low gonadotropins; failure of growth hormone to increase** (to >7 ng/mL) **after insulin-induced hypoglycemia** (to <40 mg/dL or to 50% of blood glucose level) (most common laboratory abnormality in hypopituitarism); IV TRH fails to stimulate TSH and prolactin secretion. Lytes: hyponatremia; hyperkalemia (due to decreased aldosterone). ABGs: metabolic acidosis (due to adrenal insufficiency).

Imaging Head MRI: The sella turcica shows no neoplastic or infiltrative process.

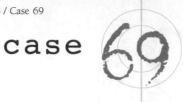

case

Sheehan Syndrome

Pathogenesis

Sheehan syndrome is a result of **ischemia following severe obstetric hemorrhage with necrosis of the anterior pituitary gland.** It is frequently associated with abruptio placentae and coagulopathy. After destruction of the pituitary gland, growth hormone, gonadotropic, thyroid, adrenal, and lactation (prolactin) functions are lost. Symptoms may be delayed for months or years.

Management

Thyroid hormone (thyroxine), **estrogen,** and **corticosteroid replacement.** Rule out obstructive pituitary tumor with MRI. Early detection is key.

Complications

Infertility, metabolic derangements, and addisonian crisis.

Breakout Point

- Sheehan syndrome is the result of pituitary necrosis, which occurs within hours of delivery and is typically preceded by postpartum hemorrhage with profound hypotension.
- There are both acute and chronic forms of Sheehan syndrome; the chronic form is more common and less severe.

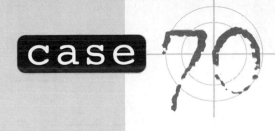

case 70

ID/CC	A 25-year-old G3P2 at 37 weeks of gestation is sent to Labor and Delivery from the clinic after ultrasound showed **estimated fetal weight at third percentile (i.e., <tenth percentile)** for gestational age.
HPI	The patient denies prenatal problems but has been noncompliant with prenatal care. She has gained 15 lbs this pregnancy and admits to **smoking** 1 pack/day throughout. She has had two prenatal visits, the last 1 month ago; the indication for ultrasound at today's visit is the lack of increase in fundal height on examination in the last month.
PE	VS: normal. Fundal height is significantly less than predicted, based on gestational age.
Labs	Group B streptococcal culture is negative.
Imaging	Abdominal ultrasound finding as above.

■ **TABLE 70-1 PREGNANCY MILESTONES OR MANEUVERS TO HELP ESTIMATE GESTATIONAL AGE**

Milestone or Maneuver	Gestational Age (wk)
Transvaginal ultrasonography–fetal heart movement	5–6
Transabdominal ultrasonography–fetal heart movement	6–7
Doppler stethoscope–fetal heart tones	10–12
Fundal height to pelvic brim	12
Perception of movement to mother ("quickening")	16–20
Conventional fetoscope–fetal heart tones	18–20
Perception of fetal movement to examiner	20
Fundal height to umbilicus	20

case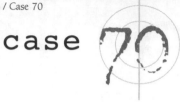

Small for Gestational Age

Pathogenesis

Small for gestational age (SGA) is defined as an infant whose **weight is less than the 10th percentile for gestational age,** and is either symmetric (all parts of the body are proportionally small) or asymmetric (some parts of the body are disproportionally small, usually small body and normal brain/skull size). It may be caused by **decreased growth potential** or **intrauterine growth restriction.** The risk of SGA increases in mothers with a previous SGA baby. Chromosomal abnormalities (trisomy 13/18/21, Turner syndrome), other congenital conditions (neural tube defects, osteogenesis imperfecta), TORCH infections (particularly CMV and rubella), and substance exposure (most commonly alcohol and cigarettes) lead to decreased growth potential. Intrauterine growth restriction is associated with maternal medical problems (hypertension, preeclampsia, renal disease, antiphospholipid syndrome, hemoglobinopathies), placental disease (causing decreased placental blood flow), malnutrition, and multiple gestation (due to earlier delivery). A fetus with decreased growth potential will be small throughout gestation; one with intrauterine growth restriction will usually fall off the growth curve.

Management

A fetus that has been consistently small throughout gestation but growing at an appropriate rate may be followed expectantly. For a fetus near term that has fallen off the growth curve, fetal testing (such as **nonstress test** and **biophysical profile**) is performed. Immediate delivery is indicated if fetal testing is nonreassuring. For SGA fetuses not near term, the risks of delivery (necessitating neonatal intensive care) are weighed against the risks of leaving the fetus in the intrauterine environment (which is causing a growth falloff).

Breakout Point

- Neonatal morbidity and mortality are more influenced by gestational age than by birthweight.
- After 20 weeks of gestation, fetal growth is followed by serial measurements of the fundal height (in cm), which should be approximately equal to gestational age (in weeks); a difference of more than 3 cm should be further evaluated with ultrasound.

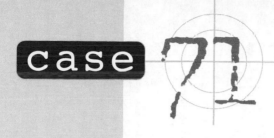

case 72

ID/CC A 28 year old primigravida at **11 weeks** gestation complains of **heavy vaginal bleeding and passage of blood clots and tissue,** with **lower abdominal pain** radiating to the back.

HPI She had **vaginal spotting** 1 week ago with mild abdominal cramps. She rested for 2 days, after which her symptoms disappeared until the onset of her present complaints. The patient brought with her to the hospital the tissue she had passed.

PE VS: normal. PE: no acute distress; mild **suprapubic tenderness;** abdomen soft with no rigidity; no rebound tenderness; uterus mildly tender and increased in size with **cervical os open.** There was minimal oozing of blood from the os and no tissue was protruding.

Labs CBC/Lytes: normal. ESR: normal; **pregnancy test positive.** UA: few RBCs. Blood type = O+.

Imaging US: uterus increased in size; **no intrauterine gestational sac;** no retained products of conception.

Gross Pathology Grossly consistent with gestational sac and products of conception.

Micro Pathology Immature placental villi and gestational sac confirmed.

OBSTETRICS

case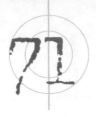

Spontaneous Abortion

Pathogenesis

The most common causes of first-trimester spontaneous abortion are **chromosomal abnormalities** (most commonly trisomies). In the second trimester, common causes include maternal anatomic defects such as bicornuate or septate uterus, Asherman syndrome (intrauterine synechiae after previous vigorous curettage), leiomyomata, incompetent cervix, placental abnormalities, drugs (cocaine, tobacco, alcohol) and toxins, and maternal illnesses such as hypothyroidism, hyperthyroidism, diabetes, SLE, and infections (toxoplasmosis, HSV, rubella, CMV).

Epidemiology

Approximately 15% to 20% of recognized pregnancies end in spontaneous abortion. Risk factors for spontaneous abortion include **multiparity, increasing age of mother and father,** and short span between pregnancies (<3 months).

Management

All couples should receive supportive counseling regarding the pregnancy loss. After three recurrent spontaneous abortions, **genetic counseling** is indicated. Administration of **RhoGAM** (Rh immune globulin) is essential to prevent Rh isoimmunization in subsequent pregnancies if the patient's blood type is Rh negative.

Complications

Retained gestational sac or placental fragments with persistent bleeding and infection, endometritis, septic shock, DIC, and uterine wall perforation during D&C.

Breakout Point

- Approximately 15% to 20% of all pregnancies end in spontaneous abortion.

■ TABLE 71-1 ABORTION TYPES (FHR = fetal heart rate)

Diagnosis	Vaginal Bleeding	Cervical Os	Tissue Passage	FHR
Missed Ab	Yes or no	Closed	No	No
Threatened Ab	Yes	Closed	No	Yes
Inevitable Ab	Yes	Open	No	Yes or no
Incomplete Ab	Yes	Open	Yes (may be protruding from os)	Usually not
Complete spontaneous Ab	Yes	Open or closed (depending on when tissue passage occurred)	Yes	No (pregnancy has already passed)

FHR: Fetal heart rate

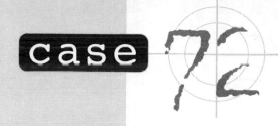

case

ID/CC A 20-year-old G1P0 at **28 weeks' gestation** by patient's stated EDD (estimated date of delivery) presents to OB triage stating "I think my water broke."

HPI Patient reports that she had a small gush of clear fluid about 5 hours prior to presentation. Since then she has had intermittent leaking of fluid, and contractions have been increasing in frequency and intensity. She reports no vaginal bleeding, and normal fetal movements. She states this had been an uncomplicated pregnancy. Aside from smoking 1/2 to 1 pack/day of cigarettes, she denies preexisting medical problems or drug use. However, the clinic where patient states she receives prenatal care **has no record of her.**

PE VS: normal. No abdominal tenderness. Fundal height measures **34 cm (size/date discrepancy).** Toco: contractions every 4 to 7 minutes, lasting 40 to 60 seconds. Fetal heart rate 130s to 140s with no decelerations, and reactive with good long-term variability. Sterile speculum examination: cervical os is **open 3 cm by visual inspection.** There is watery fluid in the posterior fornix that **turns Nitrazine paper blue.** A sample dried on a slide and viewed under a microscope shows crystalline formation upon drying (**+ pooling, + Nitrazine, + ferning =** amniotic fluid).

Labs CBC shows WBC of 14. Urinalysis is negative. Prenatal labs including HIV and hepatitis B are negative. Blood type is B Rh +. Urine toxicology screen returns positive for **methamphetamines.** A blood alcohol level that is added later is 0.

Imaging Ultrasound shows vertex presentation, estimated gestational age of 35 weeks, amniotic fluid index of 4, and biophysical profile of 6/8 (2 off for breathing).

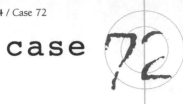

case

Substance Abuse in Pregnancy

Pathogenesis

Placental changes, carboxyhemoglobin, direct damage to fetal genes, and multiple toxic substances from **cigarette smoking** cause damage to mother and fetus (see "Complications"). How **methamphetamines** cause complications in pregnancy is not well understood, but also may be related to vasoconstriction. As a substance of abuse, methamphetamines act **powerful CNS and central and peripheral α-adrenergic and β-adrenergic receptor stimulators.** Clinically, the effects are sympathomimetic (e.g., tachycardia, diaphoresis, hyperthermia) and CNS stimulation (e.g., anorexia, euphoria, hallucinations).

Management

Social work consultation and **child protective services** referral should be made *with* the patient's knowledge. Ultrasound and prenatal labs are performed for this patient who did not receive prenatal care. A patient presenting with premature rupture of membranes (PROM) may be managed expectantly, but **indications for immediate delivery** include **fetal bradycardia, umbilical cord prolapse,** and **maternal chorioamnionitis.** Depending on the gestational age, neonatal consultation may be indicated.

Complications

Smoking during pregnancy may cause low birth weight, spontaneous abortion, stillbirth, preterm PROM, placental abruption, preterm delivery, and congenital malformations. It has also been associated with neonatal death, sudden infant death syndrome, and childhood asthma. The effects of **methamphetamine** use in pregnancy are not well known, but may include placental abruption, preterm delivery, prematurity, low birth weight, and congenital malformations including cleft lip and palate, cardiac anomalies, and CNS anomalies. Infants born to mothers abusing methamphetamines may have irritability, abnormal sleep and feeding patterns, tremors, vomiting, tachycardia, and tachypnea.

Breakout Point

- The most commonly used substances in pregnancy are cigarettes (~20%) and alcohol (10%–15%).
- Key features of fetal alcohol syndrome include growth retardation, microcephaly, small palpebral fissures, short nose, smooth philtrum, thin upper lip, cardiac defects (atrial septal defect, ventricular septal defect), and hypoplastic fifth fingernails.

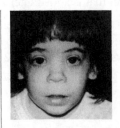

Figure 72-1. Child with fetal alcohol syndrome.

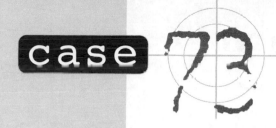

ID/CC	A 20-year-old woman complains of **amenorrhea**.
HPI	Her **last menstrual period was 10 weeks ago,** and she has had regular intercourse with her partner. She does not use contraception. Her menstrual periods have previously been regular with average flow and no dysmenorrhea. She has also noted **nausea**, especially in the morning, **fatigue,** and **increased frequency of micturition** (due to an increase in GFR).
PE	VS: BP 94/60, HR 104, afebrile. PE: **breasts full and tender with darkened areolae.** Abdominal examination is benign without masses. There is a dark line from the pubis to the umbilicus (**linea negra**). On speculum examination, the vulva, vaginal wall, and cervix are **congested and cyanotic** (CHADWICK SIGN). On bimanual examination, the **soft cervix** (GOODELL SIGN) and uterine body feel like two separate organs (because of **marked softening of the isthmus**) (HEGAR SIGN).
Labs	Pending.
Imaging	Pelvis and Abdomen as below.

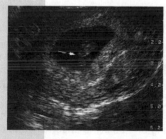

Figure 73-1. Pelvic ultrasound showing a 6-week gestation.

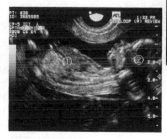

Figure 73-2. Abdominal ultrasound showing a 16-week gestation. The head (1) and abdomen (2) are indicated.

OBSTETRICS

case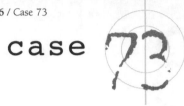

Symptoms of Early Pregnancy

Pathogenesis | Inform the patient of the pregnancy and give appropriate advice. The importance of **regular prenatal care** should be emphasized. Other major issues include **teratogen exposure** (medications, infections such as toxoplasmosis from cat litter or viral illness, and substance abuse should be surveyed), exercise, and safety/support systems. All women should be screened for **domestic violence,** because there is an increased risk of violence during pregnancy. Discuss **nutrition:** folate and iron supplementation, avoidance of unpasteurized dairy products (risk of listeria) and raw meats and fish (parasite risk), and limitation of seafood intake (mercury exposure). **Genetic counseling** with screening for diseases such as sickle cell and thalassemias, cystic fibrosis, and Tay–Sachs disease should be done if the patient's history warrants it. At initial prenatal visit order CBC, blood typing and cross-matching, rubella antibody titer, RPR/VDRL, TSH, hepatitis B surface antigen, HIV, Pap smear, cervical gonorrhea and *Chlamydia* cultures, UA for glucose and protein, urine culture, PPD, and cystic fibrosis carrier screen. Dating should also be verified by first-trimester ultrasound, which will also exclude missed abortions and ectopic pregnancies.

Breakout Point

- If pregnancy is suspected and urine pregnancy test is indeterminate, the more sensitive quantitative serum hCG assay would confirm diagnosis.
- First-trimester ultrasound should be ordered if dating or viability is uncertain, and can also be used to assess for ectopic pregnancy.

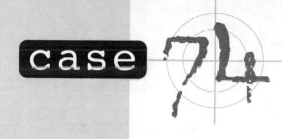

case 74

ID/CC	A 19-year-old G2P1011 delivers a **newborn** infant notable for **short long bones.**
HPI	The patient has a history of **acne** and had been taking **tetracycline** throughout the pregnancy. She did not think to mention this to her obstetrician during her pregnancy, and this history was only elicited after delivery.
PE	After birth the newborn was observed to undergo considerable **rapid compensatory bone growth.** Upon development of his **primary teeth,** these were notably **discolored** a grayish-tan color.
Labs	Not applicable.
Imaging	Not applicable.
Gross Pathology	Not applicable.
Micro Pathology	Not applicable.

case 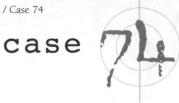74

Teratogenic Antibiotics

Pathogenesis

Tetracycline appears to **affect the calcification or hardening of bones and teeth.** This is felt to be mainly cosmetic and does not seem to affect the development of tooth enamel or cavities. Additionally, it is believed to cause **reduced growth of some bones** while the infant is being **exposed** to the medication.

Management

Tetracycline should ideally be **discontinued** prior to attempting to conceive or at least once pregnancy is diagnosed. It is important to obtain a full medical history, including current medications, at initial prenatal visits.

Complications

See "Pathogenesis."

Breakout Point

- Teratology is the study of abnormal development or the production of defects in the fetus.
- With each pregnancy there is a 3% to 5% chance of the baby being affected by a birth defect.
- The time frame from 4 to 12 weeks of gestation is the period of greatest susceptibility of the embryo to organ malformation. After this period of organogenesis, teratogens can still adversely affect organ growth and function.

■ TABLE 74-1 TERATOGENIC ANTIBIOTICS

Teratogen	Effects
Fluoroquinolones	Cartilage damage
Aminoglycosides	Ototoxicity (hearing loss), macromelia, skeletal abnormalities
Chloramphenicol	Gray baby syndrome (cardiovascular collapse)
Metronidazole	Carcinogenesis
Sulfonamides	Kernicterus

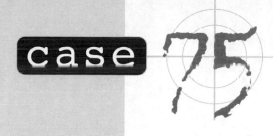

case 75

ID/CC A 32-year-old G2P1 at 41 weeks gestation is undergoing induction of labor with **oxytocin**. She complains of a **sudden**, severe, constant **abdominal pain** despite epidural anesthesia.

HPI Patient has a **history of cesarean delivery** in Guatemala 1.5 years ago; no other history of uterine surgery. She has a pfannenstiel abdominal scar (transverse incision) and an unknown uterine scar. She has been counseled extensively about the risks of a trial of labor, but refuses a cesarean delivery without a **trial of labor** (an attempted vaginal birth).

PE VS: blood pressure 70/40. Fetal heart rate is 60 (**fetal bradycardia**). Sterile vaginal examination shows **regression of the fetus** from +1 to −3 station, and her abdomen has an irregular contour that was not present earlier in labor.

Labs Not applicable.

Imaging Not applicable.

OBSTETRICS

case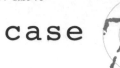

Uterine Rupture

Pathogenesis

Uterine rupture is defined as a nonsurgical complete disruption of all uterine layers, with or without bleeding and/or extrusion of part or all of the fetus or placenta. It occurs in 1% of deliveries in women with a prior cesarean section or other uterine surgery, and is most commonly associated with a classical uterine incision or a T-shaped incision. In women without prior uterine surgery, uterine rupture is rare, and may be associated with **prior abdominal trauma** (e.g., motor vehicle accident, external or internal version procedures), grand multiparity (weakens the uterine wall), and injudicious use of oxytocin. Prostaglandin cervical ripening is contraindicated in women with uterine scar because of the high incidence of uterine rupture.

Management

Uterine rupture is an **obstetric emergency,** and **immediate laparotomy** is indicated. Upon delivery, primary closure of the ruptured uterus can be done. Frequently the hysterotomy cannot be repaired, and a **total abdominal hysterectomy** is performed. If hysterectomy is not performed, future pregnancy is discouraged, as there is a significant risk for recurrent rupture; certainly, future trial of labor is contraindicated.

Complications

Uterine rupture may cause hemorrhage and hypovolemic shock. It is a major cause of maternal and fetal death.

Breakout Point

- Prostaglandin cervical ripening is contraindicated in women with uterine scars because of high incidence of uterine rupture. Careful use of oxytocin for labor augmentation, however, is allowed.
- Women with a history of more than one cesarean delivery should not labor.
- Fetal decelerations, retraction of the fetal presenting part, and sudden abdominal pain are the most common clinical manifestations.

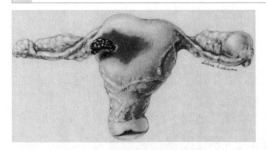

Figure 75-1. Uterine rupture.

questions

1. A 33-year-old primigravida presents for her first prenatal visit after missing her menstrual period; home pregnancy test was positive. She has no complaints, and is excited about this pregnancy. Her last menstrual period was September 6. Assuming her usual cycle length is 28 days, what is her estimated due date?

   A. May 24
   B. May 31
   C. June 6
   D. June 13
   E. June 20

2. A 16-year-old girl is accompanied by her mother to the outpatient clinic. The mother is concerned that at this age, her daughter still has not begun menstrual cycles. At quick glance, you see that the patient is approximately 5'6", is wearing a bra, and has acne on her face. Upon further questioning, she reports abdominal cramping every month; she also has a pelvic pain that has gotten worse over the past 1 to 2 months. What do you expect to see on physical examination?

   A. Webbed neck
   B. Absence of pubic and axillary hair
   C. Very bony body frame
   D. Absent uterus
   E. Hematocolpos

3. A 19-year-old college student who is not on any contraception presents "emergently" to your outpatient clinic the day after having unprotected intercourse. She is otherwise healthy, with regular menstrual cycles every 28 days; her last menstrual period was 13 days ago. She asks for advice on prevention of pregnancy, because "if I get pregnant, my mother would kill me." β-hCG is negative. After doing a physical examination, and counseling the patient on safe sex, the best option below is:

   A. Immediate dilation and curettage
   B. Reassure patient that she is not pregnant
   C. Start a daily low-dose triphasic birth control pill
   D. Levonorgestrel single dose
   E. Mifepristone

4. A 59-year-old woman with no family history of cancer was found to have microcalcifications in her left breast on routine screening mammogram. A diagnostic mammogram and ultrasound showed a 1.2-cm solid mass in the left breast. Biopsy showed invasive ductal carcinoma, estrogen receptor positive. She undergoes surgical excision with sentinel node biopsy. Surgical margins are negative, and the lymph nodes are negative. At this point, what is the most commonly recommended next step?

   A. Close follow-up with mammograms
   B. Axillary dissection
   C. Radiation
   D. Chemotherapy
   E. Radiation plus chemotherapy
   F. Mastectomy

5. A 50-year-old woman who has not seen a doctor for 3 years presents to her gynecologist for abnormal vaginal spotting. She has a history of abnormal Pap smears, but did not follow up. On examination, a 5-cm cervical mass is palpated, with involvement of the right parametrium. Rectal examination shows that the tumor also extends to the rectum. Biopsy of the cervical mass shows poorly differentiated squamous cell carcinoma. The patient is otherwise healthy, without significant comorbidities. PET/CT shows no distant metastasis. What is the appropriate treatment?

   A. Radical hysterectomy
   B. Radical hysterectomy, chemotherapy
   C. Radical hysterectomy, chemotherapy, radiation
   D. Radical hysterectomy, radiation
   E. Chemotherapy and radiation

6. A 60-year-old postmenopausal woman presents with vaginal spotting. She did use hormonal replacement therapy for about 3 years for hot flashes, but stopped 1 year ago because of concerns that it increases the risk of endometrial cancer. Examination shows old blood in the vagina, a normal-sized uterus, and normal parametria. Transvaginal ultrasound shows thickened endometrium, which is biopsy-proven adenocarcinoma. Chest CT shows there is no distant metastasis.

   The patient is taken for TAHBSO and surgical staging by the gynecologic oncologist. Pathology shows endometrial adenocarcinoma invading <1/2 of the myometrium, without cervical involvement. Peritoneal washing, ovaries, fallopian tubes are all negative. One right pelvic node is positive, out of 25 nodes taken. What is the stage of this disease?

A. IB
B. II
C. IIIA
D. IIIB
E. IIIC

7. A 26-year-old petit primigravida at 38 weeks' gestation has been in labor for 10 hours. Membranes are ruptured. Prior to the onset of labor, there was suspicion of cephalopelvic disproportion based on pelvimetry and fetal size, but the decision was made to attempt vaginal delivery. Examination shows cervix is dilated at 7 cm, and the fetus in occiput anterior position, at −1 station. Progression of labor has been protracted throughout, and the mother is noticeably fatigued. Fetal heart tracing is reassuring, and contractions are regular at every 3 minutes. The most appropriate management at this time is:

A. Cesarean section
B. Magnesium sulfate tocolysis to allow the mother to rest
C. Oxytocin administration
D. Fetal extraction with vacuum
E. Rotating the fetus to an occiput posterior position

8. A 23-year-old woman presents to the Ob/Gyn for annual checkup. She has a new boyfriend of 1 month and uses a diaphragm as means of contraception. Review of systems is entirely negative, and a thorough physical examination only reveals mildly inflamed cervix. Pap smear is performed, showing normal endocervical cells, but gonorrhea/ *Chlamydia* probes come back positive for gonorrhea. Appropriate treatment is:

A. Ceftriaxone
B. Doxycycline
C. Sexual partner should be identified and treated
D. Repeat Pap smear
E. Ceftriaxone and doxycycline

9. A 23-year-old G2P0 at 34 weeks' gestation is found to have a blood pressure of 170/115 on a routine visit. Repeat blood pressure check the next day confirms this reading. Her prior systolic blood pressures have been in the 130s. Urine dipstick shows 3+ protein. Her liver function tests and CBC are normal, and she denies seizures. She does exhibit edema in the hands and face, and reports headaches with visual changes. What is the most appropriate management?

A. Urinalysis to check for proteinuria
B. Maintain high blood pressure to insure sufficient perfusion pressure for fetus
C. Immediate imaging of the head to check for hemorrhage
D. Emergency cesarean section
E. Magnesium sulfate, hydralazine, dexamethasone; delivery upon patient stabilization

10. A 28-year-old G2P1 at 36 weeks' gestation presents for a routine prenatal visit. Her previous child was born via a planned cesarean section, using a low transverse incision. However, the postpartum course was complicated by bacteremia, requiring IV antibiotics and a 2-week hospitalization. She also experienced significant pain at the incision. The current pregnancy has been uncomplicated, and the patient is otherwise healthy without history of other abdominal surgery. Ultrasound estimates the fetus to weigh 3,500 g. The patient requests an attempt of vaginal delivery. Which of the following statements is most correct?

A. Vaginal delivery is contraindicated after previous cesarean section.
B. Oxytocin should be used to hasten delivery, and minimize risk of uterine rupture.
C. The chance of uterine rupture from vaginal delivery in this case is 1%.
D. After prior cesarean section, vaginal delivery is contraindicated because of fetal size >3,000 g.
E. Calcium channel blockers should be given during labor to decrease the strength of uterine contractions.

11. A 65-year-old woman presents with several months of vaginal burning, pruritis, and occasional nonodorous yellow discharge. She also reports occasional mild dysuria. The patient denies fever or vaginal bleeding. She has tried over-the-counter antifungal creams, with mixed results. Examination shows scant pubic hair, nonedematous vulva with decreased elasticity, and dry vaginal epithelium, without obvious lesions. After doing the proper workup, the treatment for the most likely diagnosis is:

A. Clindamycin
B. Oral fluconazole
C. Doxycycline
D. Topical estrogen
E. Metronidazole

12. A 35-year-old G6P3 at 36 weeks' gestation arrives at the Emergency Department by ambulance with painless vaginal bleeding worsening over the past hour. She has had a few episodes of vaginal spotting over the past several weeks, but because of the self-limited nature of these episodes, has largely ignored them and not told her obstetrician. Upon examination, you see a pale woman with heart rate of 110 and blood pressure of 90/50. Based on the history and presentation, you suspect that the patient may have placenta previa. Which of the following should be the next step in this obstetric emergency?

A. Digital vaginal examination to find the source of bleeding
B. Ultrasound to make the diagnosis
C. IV fluids
D. Stool guaiac
E. Cesarean section delivery

13. A 55-year-old postmenopausal woman presents to your clinic reporting intolerable hot flashes. She has tried SSRIs, gabapentin, and even alternative therapies without significant benefit, and asks about hormone replacement therapy (HRT). She has read about HRT, and understands that there is an increased risk of breast cancer and "blood clots." The patient is otherwise healthy, except for hypertension and mild hypercholesterolemia, but is without previous cancers or thromboembolic disease. Which of the following is a contraindication of hormonal replacement therapy with combined estrogen and progestin?

A. Coronary artery disease
B. Osteoporosis
C. Colorectal cancer
D. Severe hot flash symptoms
E. Vaginal atrophy

14. A 33-year-old pregnant woman presents with 3 days of dysuria and urinary frequency. She reports no fever, chills, urethral discharge, and has no costovertebral angle pain on examination. Urinalysis shows >5 WBCs/high-power field, and is positive for nitrites and leukocyte esterase. You send the urine for culture and sensitivities, and give the patient a prescription for empiric treatment. Which of the following antibiotics is most appropriate?

A. Topical antibiotic only
B. Levofloxacin
C. Bactrim (TMP-SMX)
D. Amoxicillin
E. Doxycycline

15. A 25-year-old G1P1 reports right breast tenderness, and low-grade fevers to 99.5°F. She had a vaginal delivery of a healthy boy 3 weeks ago, after an uncomplicated pregnancy, and is breast-feeding. On examination, an area of the right breast, at 9:00 from the nipple, is erythematous, hard, warm, and tender to touch. Which of the following represents proper immediate management of this scenario?

    A. Cessation of breast-feeding until infection is resolved
    B. Empiric antibiotic treatment with dicloxacillin
    C. Mammogram to rule out inflammatory breast cancer
    D. Skin biopsy
    E. Incision and drainage

16. A 33-year-old G5P1, last menstrual period 10 weeks ago, presents to the Emergency Department with vaginal bleeding and mild abdominal cramping for 12 hours. She reports having passed quarter-sized "clots." On examination, the cervix is open, and tissue is seen in the vagina. Serum β-hCG level is 5,000. Ultrasound shows no fetal heartbeat. Which of the following is the most accurate description of this scenario?

    A. Threatened abortion
    B. Therapeutic abortion
    C. Inevitable abortion
    D. Incomplete abortion
    E. Missed abortion

17. A 28-year-old primigravida at 41 weeks' gestation is on the Labor and Delivery floor, and now has contractions about every 5 minutes. Her pregnancy has been uncomplicated throughout. You are checking on the patient, and look through the tocometer and fetal heart tracing. If seen, which of the following patterns on the tracing would be most concerning?

    A. No decelerations
    B. Decelerations beginning and ending with contractions
    C. Occasional sharp drop in fetal heart rate, which quickly returns to baseline
    D. Decelerations beginning after contractions start and ending after contractions end
    E. Fetal heart rate rising as high as 160

18. A 34-year-old woman presents for a routine postpartum follow-up. She has a history of 2 miscarriages, 1 therapeutic abortion, a twin birth at term, and 2 singleton births at term. What is her gravida and parity?

A. G6P4-1-1-3
B. G6P3-0-3-4
C. G6P2-1-2-1
D. G6P2-1-3-4
E. G6P2-2-4-3

19. A 30-year-old primigravida at 36 weeks' gestation presents to Labor and Delivery with onset of contractions. She reports good fetal movement, and no leakage of fluid or vaginal bleeding. Contractions are irregular in timing (ranging between every 2 to >10 minutes), duration, and intensity. Leopold maneuver shows vertex fetal position. Sterile vaginal examination shows a closed cervix with no pooled fluid in the vagina. Fetal heart rate monitor shows heart rate in the 140s with a reactive nonstress test. What is the appropriate assessment and plan?

A. Patient is not in labor, discharge to home
B. Patient is in early labor, discharge to home
C. Patient is in early labor, admit to Labor and Delivery
D. Patient is in early labor, but irregular contractions are concerning. Admit and give magnesium sulfate for tocolysis.
E. Patient is in early labor, but irregular contractions are concerning. Prepare for cesarean section.

20. A 33-year-old P2N0 presents for routine prenatal care during the third trimester and is found to have a hemoglobin of 11.5. The patient is otherwise healthy and has no previous history of anemia. She has had an uncomplicated pregnancy. On review of systems, she denies gross hematuria or hematochezia. She takes a prenatal vitamin daily. Vital signs are within normal limits. What is the appropriate next step in the workup?

A. Coagulation studies, PT/PTT/INR
B. Rectal examination for occult blood
C. Blood transfusion
D. Serum folate level
E. No further workup

answers

1-D

A. The formula for calculating due date for a woman with 28-day menstrual cycle is: date of last menstrual period −3 months +7 days. May 24 [Incorrect] is not the correct estimated due date according to this equation.

B. The formula for calculating due date for a woman with 28-day menstrual cycle is: date of last menstrual period −3 months +7 days. May 31 [Incorrect] is not the correct estimated due date according to this equation.

C. The formula for calculating due date for a woman with 28-day menstrual cycle is: date of last menstrual period −3 months +7 days. June 6 [Incorrect] is not the correct estimated due date according to this equation.

D. The formula for calculating due date for a woman with 28-day menstrual cycle is: date of last menstrual period −3 months +7 days. In this case, last menstrual period of September 6 would correspond to a June 13 [Correct] due date. If the menstrual cycle length is not 28 days, add or subtract the difference in cycle length to the previously estimated date. For example, if the cycle length is 31 days, the estimated due date would be June 16.

E. The formula for calculating due date for a woman with 28-day menstrual cycle is: date of last menstrual period − 3 months +7 days. June 20 [Incorrect] is not the correct estimated due date according to this equation.

2-E

A. Turner syndrome (45 XO) is characterized by short stature and webbed neck [Incorrect]. The amenorrhea is due to gonadal dysgenesis; by puberty there are usually no primordial oocytes in the ovaries.

B. Absence of pubic and axillary hair [Incorrect] would be the case for androgen insensitivity. On physical examination, would also see the vagina ending in a blind pouch. The patient's monthly cramping makes this diagnosis unlikely.

C. Anorexia nervosa (very bony body frame) [Incorrect] may cause functional hypothalamic amenorrhea but is not consistent with the presentation of this case.

D. Absent uterus [Incorrect] is also a cause of primary amenorrhea but is not consistent with this case.

E. The patient's symptoms are consistent with imperforate hymen. She has begun puberty—given her height, breast development, and acne—and the key to this case is that her monthly cramping indicates menstruation, thus making other causes of primary amenorrhea unlikely. The worsening pelvic pain is from buildup of blood behind the hymen (hematocolpos) [Correct], which is easily seen on physical examination. Treatment is surgical.

3-D

A. Immediate D&C [Incorrect] is not indicated—and would be ineffective—because implantation has not yet taken place.

B. Negative hCG rules out pregnancy before starting therapy, but does not rule out possible fertilization of ovum from unprotected intercourse 1 day prior to the test. Therefore, reassuring the patient she is not pregnant [Incorrect] would not be the best option.

C. A minimum of 100 μg of ethinyl estradiol in two divided doses needs to be given to be effective. Also, estradiol-containing regimens cause more nausea/vomiting than levonorgestrel. Therefore, starting a daily low-dose triphasic birth control pill [Incorrect] is not the best option.

D. "Emergency contraception" in the form of Plan B (levonorgestrel) is approved by the FDA and is available over-the-counter without prescription for women aged 18 and older. Plan B contains 2 pills of levonorgestrel, 0.75 mg each, to be taken 12 hours apart. A single 1.5-mg dose of levonorgestrel [Correct] has been proven to be equally efficacious. Side effects of levonorgestrel may include nausea and vomiting. Treatment should start as soon as possible, but may be started within 120 hours of unprotected intercourse. Immediate implantation of a copper intrauterine device is also effective, and provides continued contraception after the initial event.

E. Mifepristone (RU-486) [Incorrect], an antiprogestin, is also efficacious as an emergency contraceptive. It can inhibit implantation as well as ovulation. However, it is not approved in the United States for this indication.

4-C

A. Radiation therapy is needed after breast-conserving therapy. Therefore, close follow-up with mammograms [Incorrect] alone represents inadequate treatment.

B. Axillary dissection [Incorrect] is not necessary if sentinel nodes are negative.

C. The patient has stage I disease. The standard of care is breast-conserving surgery (i.e., lumpectomy) followed by radiation [Correct], or mastectomy alone; the two options are deemed equivalent in the cure rates. Mastectomy is the much less commonly chosen option, especially for a woman without family history of breast cancer. For ER-positive tumor, the patient will need hormonal therapy (e.g., tamoxifen), but that is usually given after radiation is finished, and is not the next step.

D. Chemotherapy [Incorrect] is not indicated for stage I disease. The possible benefit, especially with ER-positive cancer, is too small when weighed against possible side effects.

E. Mastectomy [Incorrect], followed by hormonal therapy is also a reasonable option. Radiation would not be necessary in this case. However, this is not the most commonly recommended treatment modality.

5-E

A. Surgical treatment in this case would involve pelvic exenteration (i.e., an en-bloc resection of the female reproductive organs, lower urinary tract, and part of the rectosigmoid) to obtain clear margins. This is a very morbid procedure, and is done usually as a "last-ditch" curative effort when there are no other options. Radical hysterectomy [Incorrect] alone would be an inadequate surgical procedure in this case.

B. Radical hysterectomy [Incorrect] would be an inadequate surgical procedure in this case, even with the addition of chemotherapy.

C. Radical hysterectomy [Incorrect] would be an inadequate surgical procedure in this case, even with the addition of chemotherapy and radiation.

D. Radical hysterectomy [Incorrect] would be an inadequate surgical procedure in this case, even with the addition of radiation.

E. The patient has FIGO stage IVA disease, because of rectal involvement. For stage IIB-IVA cervical cancer, the most common treatment recommended is concurrent chemotherapy and radiation [Correct], which has excellent cure rates.

6-E

A. IB [Incorrect]: Tumor confined to the uterus and invades to <1/2 thickness of the myometrium.

B. II [Incorrect]: Tumor invades the cervix but is confined to the uterus/cervix.

C. IIIA [Incorrect]: Tumor involves uterine serosa and/or adnexa. Or positive peritoneal washings.

D. IIIB [Incorrect]: Tumor involves the vagina.

E. FIGO staging for endometrial cancer is based on surgical findings. Any positive pelvic or para-aortic node makes it stage IIIC [Correct] disease, irrespective of how many positive nodes are found. (Note: on the other hand, FIGO staging for cervical cancer does not take nodal status into account).

7-A

A. A common cause of protracted or arrested labor is cepahlopelvic discordance (CPD)—disproportion between the sizes of the mother's pelvis and the fetus. Because a clinician's ability to predict CPD is poor, even with pelvimetry, vaginal delivery is often attempted. In general, when protracted or arrested labor is encountered, the decision regarding whether to perform cesarean section is made on an individual basis. In this case, because CPD is the cause, continued vaginal delivery would not be appropriate. The patient's fatigue from prolonged labor—and likely inability to deliver on her own—is another strong indication for cesarean section [Correct].

B. Magnesium sulfate tocolysis [Incorrrect] is often used to halt preterm labor. It is not appropriate in this case.

C. Oxytocin [Incorrect] may be given to augment labor when protraction or arrest occurs during the first stage. However, it is contraindicated in CPD.

D. Fetal extraction with vacuum or forceps [Incorrect] may be used for protraction or arrest during the second stage of labor.

E. The fetus is in occiput anterior position, which is the most favorable position for delivery. Rotating the fetus to an occiput posterior position [Incorrect] is not helpful.

8-E

A. Treatment for gonorrhea includes ceftriaxone or fluoroquinolones. However, women should also be treated for possible concomitant *Chlamydia* with doxycycline or azithromycin, because *Chlamydia* is more often missed on testing. Therefore, ceftriaxone [Incorrect] alone would not be an appropriate treatment.

B. Women testing positive for gonorrhea should also be treated for possible concomitant *Chlamydia* with doxycycline or azithromycin, because *Chlamydia* is more often missed on testing. Doxycycline [Incorrect] alone would not be an appropriate treatment.

C. Sexual partners should be identified and also treated [Incorrect]; however, this is not an appropriate treatment for the patient's gonorrhea.

D. Repeat Pap smear [Incorrect] is not necessary because initial results were normal.

E. Up to 50% to 80% of women with gonorrhea are asymptomatic, as is the woman in this case. Treatment for gonorrhea includes ceftriaxone or fluoroquinolones. Women should also be treated for possible concomitant *Chlamydia* with doxycycline or azithromycin, because *Chlamydia* is more often missed on testing. Ceftriaxone and doxycycline [Correct] would be the appropriate treatment.

9-E

A. Urine dipstick already shows 3+ protein; urinalysis to confirm proteinuria [Incorrect] is not necessary.

B. Elevated blood pressure should be lowered appropriately, not maintained at high levels [Incorrect].

C. Immediate imaging of the head to check for hemorrhage [Incorrect] should not be performed at this time.

D. Once the patient is stable, immediate delivery is indicated if the fetus is of viable age. Usually, vaginal delivery is attempted (via induction); emergency cesarean section [Incorrect] is not necessary.

E. The patient in this case has preeclampsia, the diagnosis of which requires elevated blood pressure (>140/90) and proteinuria. Having *any* of the following symptoms makes it "severe preeclampsia": BP >160/110, 3–4+ protein on dipstick, or associated symptoms such as headache, visual changes, altered consciousness, epigastric or right upper quadrant abdominal pain, liver function tests >2 × normal, oliguria, pulmonary edema, or significant thrombocytopenia (platelets <100,000). Management of preeclampsia is to stabilize the patient first, with seizure prophylaxis (most commonly magnesium sulfate) and lowering of blood pressure (hydralazine is a direct arteriolar dilator). Dexamethasone [Correct] is given to hasten fetal lung maturity. Once the patient is stable, immediate delivery is indicated if the fetus is of viable age.

10-C

A. The patient in this case had a low transverse incision, so is a candidate for labor. Vaginal delivery is not contraindicated [Incorrect] in this case.

B. Oxytocin [Incorrect] increases the risk of uterine rupture in women with prior cesarean section, but may be used with caution, if necessary.

C. Uterine rupture, an obstetric emergency with significant mortality risk to both the mother and fetus, is the primary concern for women attempting vaginal delivery after prior cesarean section(s). Women with one prior cesarean section via low transverse incision or low uterine vertical incision are candidates for trial of labor, with a low risk of rupture of ~1% or less [Correct]. Patients with classical uterine incision or a T-shaped incision, or more than one prior cesarean section, should not attempt labor, as the risk of uterine rupture is significantly higher.

D. There is no evidence that a fetus >3,000 g [Incorrect] increases the risk of uterine rupture.

E. There is no evidence that calcium channel blockers [Incorrect] decrease the risk of uterine rupture.

11-D

A. Bacterial vaginosis, for which clindamycin [Incorrect] is the appropriate treatment, is characterized by profuse discharge with a characteristic "fishy" smell. Diagnosis is made by wet prep of vaginal swab, revealing "clue" cells.

B. Oral or topical antifungals (such as oral fluconazole) [Incorrect] are appropriate treatments for vaginal yeast infections. Diagnosis may be made by viewing the KOH prep of vaginal discharge under the microscope, and seeing the characteristic branching hyphae and spores. This is the less likely diagnosis in this case because the patient has already tried antifungal creams, without success.

C. *Chlamydia*, for which doxycycline [Incorrect] is the appropriate treatment, is an STD and is an uncommon diagnosis is this age group.

D. The most likely diagnosis in this scenario is atrophic vaginitis, which can present with all of the stated symptoms. The cause is chronic low estrogen levels, leading to dryness and inflammation of the vagina, with thinning of the epithelium. Treatment is with lubricants or moisturizers for mild symptoms; vaginal estrogen [Correct] is also effective and results in minimal systemic absorption.

E. Metronidazole [Incorrect] may be used to treat bacterial vaginosis or *Trichomonas vaginalis*. *Trichomonas* is also an STD and is characterized by profuse malodorous discharge. The classic "strawberry" appearance of the cervix occurs only in about 10% of cases. Wet prep shows the protozoa.

12-C

A. Digital examination is [Incorrect] contraindicated for suspected placenta previa, as it may worsen bleeding. Careful speculum examination is the preferred method.

B. Ultrasound [Incorrect] is the best way to make a definitive diagnosis of placenta previa, but should not be performed before stabilizing the patient.

C. In obstetric emergencies, like any other medical emergency, ABCs (airway, breathing, circulation) should always be performed first. The patient should receive oxygen and IV fluid resuscitation [Correct]. Type and cross should be sent in preparation for blood transfusion. After the patient is stabilized, then appropriate treatment for the specific condition should begin. Any woman presenting during the third trimester with painless bright-red bleeding should be thought of as having placenta previa until proven otherwise. Treatment involves pelvic rest and conservative management (i.e., observation) until the fetus is viable; then elective cesarean section may be considered. However, if the bleeding is severe (like in this case), patient should undergo emergency cesarean section after initial stabilization. If the fetus is <34 weeks' gestation, betamethasone should be given to hasten fetal lung maturation.

D. The bleeding is vaginal and there is no reason to suspect a second source of bleeding. Stool guaiac [Incorrect] would not be the next step in this obstetric emergency.

E. After patient stabilization, emergency cesarean delivery [Incorrect] is required.

13-A

A. HRT is commonly given as a combination of estrogen and progestin. Unopposed estrogen should not be used for HRT because of increased risk of endometrial hyperplasia and cancer, except for women with previous hysterectomy. There are many potential benefits of HRT, as listed, except for coronary artery disease [Correct] prevention. The Women's Health Study has shown that combined therapy may actually slightly increase the risk of coronary artery disease. Alternative therapies for postmenopausal women may include calcium with vitamin D and exercise for bone health, and topical estrogen (which has minimal systemic absorption) to prevent vaginal atrophy.

B. Osteoporosis [Incorrect], severe hot flash symptoms, and vaginal atrophy are all indications for HRT.

C. There is no evidence that colorectal cancer [Incorrect] is exacerbated by HRT.

D. Osteoporosis, severe hot flash symptoms [Incorrect], and vaginal atrophy are all indications for HRT.

E. Osteoporosis, severe hot flash symptoms, and vaginal atrophy [Incorrect] are all indications for HRT.

14-D

A. Topical antibiotic treatment [Incorrect] would not be sufficient treatment for UTI.

B. The use of quinolones during pregnancy is not well studied. However, animal studies have shown decreased body weight and increased fetal mortality. Therefore, levofloxacin [Incorrect] is not recommended as first-line treatment during pregnancy.

C. Sulfonamides, such as Bactrim (TMP-SMX) [Incorrect], increase the risk of kernicterus in the newborn, and should not be used during the third trimester.

D. During pregnancy, because of smooth muscle relaxation from progesterone effect, and mechanical compression from an enlarged uterus causing vesicoureteral reflux, there is a higher incidence of ascending urinary tract infections. Therefore, pregnant women are screened for asymptomatic bacteriuria; even for those without symptoms of the patient in this case, systemic antibiotic treatment would be indicated. *E. coli* is the most common causative organism of UTIs. In this case, the patient exhibits no symptom for pyelonephritis and has cystitis. Common antibiotics used include quinolones (such as levofloxacin), Bactrim, amoxicillin, doxycycline, and also cephalosporins. Of the choices listed, amoxicillin [Correct] is the safest during pregnancy; cephalosporins (e.g., ceftriaxone) would be another good choice.

E. Doxycycline [Incorrect] is a tetracycline derivative. When given during second or third trimester, both cause permanent yellow discoloration of the teeth.

15-B

A. Women should continue to breast-feed, which would prevent intraductal accumulation of infectious material. Cessation of breast-feeding until infection is resolved [Incorrect] would not be proper management of this scenario.

B. Mastitis occurs in 1% to 3% of lactating women, and is a local infection most commonly caused by *Staphylococcus aureus*, *Streptococcus*, or *E. coli*. It should be differentiated from normal breast engorgement in lactating women, which is characterized by diffusely warm and tender breasts. Treatment includes an anti-inflammatory (such as ibuprofen) for pain control, and antibiotic such as dicloxacillin [Correct] for 10 to 14 days. In some cases it may progress to formation of an abscess, which would require treatment with incision and drainage.

C. Although inflammatory breast cancer [Incorrect] may present similarly (with enlarged, firm, and tender breast, and also associated skin changes), there is no reason to suspect breast cancer in this case, and breast cancer would be very rare in a 25-year-old woman.

D. Skin biopsy [Incorrect] is not indicated in this case when the clinical diagnosis of mastitis is made. Such workup may be required if empiric treatment fails to resolve the presenting symptoms.

E. Incision and drainage [Incorrect] would not represent proper immediate management of this scenario.

16-D

A. May or may not progress to spontaneous abortion. Threatened abortion [Incorrect] is usually characterized by vaginal bleeding but closed cervix.

B. Therapeutic abortion [Incorrect] is an elective procedure ending pregnancy.

C. Inevitable abortion [Incorrect], which will progress to spontaneous abortion, is a condition characterized by profuse vaginal bleeding and an open cervix.

D. The case described is a "spontaneous abortion," or miscarriage, which can occur up to 20 weeks' gestation; after that, it is called "preterm delivery." "Incomplete abortion" [Correct] describes a miscarriage when not all of the products of conception have exited the body, as opposed to "complete abortion."

E. Missed abortion [Incorrect] is a miscarriage with retention of an abortus in the uterus.

17-D

A. No fetal heart rate deceleration [Incorrect] with contraction is a normal finding.

B. Decelerations beginning and ending with contractions [Incorrect] describes early decelerations, which are thought to be due to fetal head compression.

C. Occasional sharp drop in fetal heart rate, which quickly returns to baseline [Incorrect], describes variable decelerations, which are due to umbilical cord compression.

D. Decelerations beginning after contractions start and ending after contractions end [Correct] describes late decelerations, which are due to uteroplacental insufficiency. The resultant hypoxia leads to fetal shunting of blood to vital organs (e.g., brain, heart, placenta) via constriction of peripheral arteries; the hypertension from arterial constriction activates baroreceptors, which leads to vagal stimulation of the fetal heart and the lowering of heart rate. Late decelerations are a worrisome sign and may progress to fetal bradycardia.

E. Fetal heart rate should be between 110 and 160. Fetal heart rate rising as high as 160 [Incorrect] is a normal finding.

18-B

A. G6P4-1-1-3 [Incorrect] indicates the incorrect number of term deliveries, preterm deliveries, abortuses, and living children.

B. Gravida refers to how many times a woman has been pregnant. Parity refers to the number of pregnancies resulting in birth beyond 20 weeks' gestation, or infants weighing more than 500 g. Parity is further divided into number of pregnancies resulting in term deliveries (over 37 weeks), number of pregnancies resulting in preterm deliveries, number of abortuses, and number of living children. Therefore, in this case, the woman is G6 (6 pregnancies), P3 (3 term deliveries) – 0 (no preterm deliveries) – 3 (3 abortuses) – 4 (4 living children) [Correct].

C. G6P2-1-2-1[Incorrect] indicates the incorrect number of term deliveries, preterm deliveries, abortuses, and living children.

D. G6P2-1-3-4 [Incorrect] indicates the incorrect number of term deliveries, preterm deliveries, abortuses, and living children.

E. G6P2-2-4-3 [Incorrect] indicates the incorrect number of term deliveries, preterm deliveries, abortuses, and living children.

19-A

    A. "Labor" is defined as contractions that cause cervical change. The described symptoms in this case are consistent with "false labor," which is characterized by irregular contractions that do not lead to cervical change. The patient is understandably anxious with this first pregnancy, but proper management is reassurance and further teaching about the signs and symptoms of labor. Patient should be discharged to home [Correct].

    B. The patient is not in early labor [Incorrect].

    C. The patient is not in early labor [Incorrect]. The described symptoms in this case are consistent with "false labor." Admission is not indicated.

    D. The patient is not in early labor [Incorrect]. The described symptoms in this case are consistent with "false labor." Admission is not indicated.

    E. The patient is not in early labor [Incorrect]. Cesarean section is not indicated because the patient is in "false labor."

20-E

    A. Coagulation studies [Incorrect] would not be performed in this case because there is no reason to suspect abnormal bleeding.

    B. Rectal examination for occult blood [Incorrect] would not be performed in this case because there is no reason to suspect abnormal bleeding.

    C. Blood transfusion [Incorrect] is not given because her hemoglobin is normal.

    D. Serum folate level [Incorrect] would not be obtained in this case, because she has a normal hemoglobin and takes a prenatal vitamin that contains folate.

    E. The woman in this case has a hemoglobin of 11.5, so no further workup is necessary. During pregnancy, plasma volume increases by up to 50%, but red blood cell volume increases only by 20% to 30%. Therefore, anemia during pregnancy is a physiologic phenomenon, and "normal" hemoglobin values for a woman in third trimester are between 11 and 12 g/dL. On the other hand, approximately 1% of pregnancies are complicated by megaloblastic anemia, which is usually caused by serum folate deficiency.

credits

Berek JS. *Berek & Novak's Gynecology*. 14th ed. Philadelphia: Lippincott Williams & Wilkins; 2005. Figs. 10.4 (28-1), 10.6 (28-2), 6.49 (39-1).

Bhushan V, Le T, Pall V. *Underground Clinical Vignettes: Step 2 Obstetrics & Gynecology*. 3rd ed. Malden, MA: Blackwell; 2005. Figs. 10 (9-1), 26A&B (22-1), 17A (26-1), 17B (26-2), 17C (26-3), 3A (33-1), 3B (33-2), 41 (49-1), 35 (57-1), 40A (73-1), 40B (73-2).

Cohen WR. *Cherry & Merkatz's Complications of Pregnancy*. 5th ed. Baltimore: Lippincott Williams & Wilkins; 2000. Table 51-1 (63-1).

Eisenberg RL. *Clinical Imaging: An Atlas of Differential Diagnosis*. 4th ed. Philadelphia: Lippincott Williams & Wilkins; 2002. Fig. C43-4A&B (67-1).

Emans SJ, Laufer MR, Goldstein DP. *Pediatric and Adolescent Gynecology*. 5th ed. Philadelphia: Lippincott Williams & Wilkins; 2004. Figs. 17.6 (5-1), 9.5 (16-1).

Fiebach NH, et al. *Principles of Ambulatory Medicine*. 7th ed. Baltimore: Lippiincott Williams & Wilkins; 2007. Table 102.1 (3-1).

Gorbach SL, Bartlett JG, Blacklow NR. *Infectious Diseases*. 3rd ed. Philadelphia: Lippincott Williams & Wilkins; 2003. Fig. 103.1 (10-1).

Goroll AH, et al. *Primary Care Medicine: Office Evaluation and Management of the Adult Patient*. 5th ed. Philadelphia: Lippincott Williams & Wilkins; 2006. Table 133.1 (31-1).

Hall JC. *Sauer's Manual of Skin Disorders*. 9th ed. Philadelphia: Lippincott Williams & Wilkins; 2006. Fig. 22-3E (24-1).

Hou MY, MD. Beth Israel Deaconess Medical Center, Boston MA. 2005. Courtesy Figs. (29-1A&B).

Humes DH, ed. *Kelley's Textbook of Internal Medicine*. 4th ed. Philadelphia: Lippincott Williams & Wilkins; 2000. Table 458.2 (30-1).

Loeser JD, Butler SH, et al. *Bonica's Management of Pain*. 3rd ed. Philadelphia: Lippincott Williams & Wilkins; 2000. Fig. 83-1 (8-1).

McMillan JA, Fergin RD, et al. *Oski's Pediatrics: Principles and Practice.* 4th ed. Philadelphia: Lippincott Williams & Wilkins; 2006. Fig. from Appendix B (72-1).

Mulholland MW, Lillemoe KD, Doherty GM, et al. *Greenfield's Surgery: Scientific Principles & Practice.* 4th ed. Philadelphia: Lippincott Williams & Wilkins; 2005. Fig. 76.19 (36-1).

Rock JA, Jones HW III. *Te Linde's Operative Gynecology.* 9th ed. Philadelphia: Lippincott Williams & Wilkins; 2003. Fig. 20.15 (75-1).

Scott JR, Gibbs RS, et al. *Danforth's Obstetrics and Gynecology.* 9th ed. Philadelphia: Lippincott Williams & Wilkins; 2003. Figs. 22.10 (44-1), 21.1 (45-1), 9.4 (47-1), 3.1 (51-1), 4.5 (56-1), 17.1 (58-1), 45.2 (59-1), 20.6 (60-1), 1.1 (65-1); Tables 32.2 (4-1), 38.1 (11-1), 36.2 (18-1), 57.3 (35-1), 25.6 (43-1), 31.8 (50-1), 19.5 (64-1), 10.6 (66-1).

Taylor RB. *Annual of Family Practice.* 2nd ed. Philadelphia: Lippincott Williams & Wilkins; 2003. Table 14.4.5 (70-1).

Wolfson AB, et al. *Harwood-Nuss' Clinical Practice of Emergency Medicine.* 4th ed. Baltimore: Lippincott Williams & Wilkins; 2005. Tables 94.2 (17-1), 94.4 (55-1).

case list

GYNECOLOGY

1. Bacterial Vaginosis
2. Bartholin Cyst
3. Candidal Vaginitis
4. Cervicitis
5. Condylomata Acuminata
6. Contraception
7. Dysfunctional Uterine Bleeding
8. Dysmenorrhea
9. Endometriosis
10. Gonorrhea
11. Infertility
12. Meigs Syndrome
13. Menopause
14. Pelvic Inflammatory Disease
15. Pelvic Tuberculosis
16. Polycystic Ovarian Disease
17. Postcoital Bleeding (Benign Endocervical Polyp)
18. Premenstrual Dysphoric Disorder
19. Primary Amenorrhea—Androgen Insensitivity
20. Primary Amenorrhea (Turner Syndrome)
21. Rape/Sexual Assault
22. Secondary Amenorrhea (Prolactinoma)
23. Side Effects of Oral Contraception
24. Syphilis
25. Tanner Stages
26. Teratoma
27. Staphylococcal Toxic Shock Syndrome
28. Tubal Ligation
29. Tubo ovarian Abscess
30. Urinary Incontinence
31. Urinary Tract Infection

GYNECOLOGIC ONCOLOGY

32. Bloody Breast Discharge
33. Breast Cancer
34. Cervical Cancer
35. Hydatidiform Mole/Choriocarcinoma
36. Ductal Carcinoma in Situ
37. Ovarian Cancer
38. Postmenopausal Bleeding (Uterine Cancer)
39. Uterine Fibroids
40. Vaginal Cancer
41. Vulvar Cancer

OBSTETRICS

42. Acute Fatty Liver of Pregnancy
43. Amniotic Fluid Embolism
44. Arrested Labor
45. Breech Presentation
46. Chorioamnionitis
47. Deceleration of Fetal Heart Rate
48. Eclampsia
49. Ectopic Pregnancy
50. Elective Abortion
51. Epidural Anesthesia During Labor
52. Gestational Diabetes
53. HELLP Syndrome
54. HIV Transmission in Pregnancy
55. Hyperemesis Gravidarum
56. Incompetent Cervix

index